39.50

Portal Hypertension II

Portal Hypertension II

Proceedings of the
Second Baveno International Consensus Workshop
on Definitions, Methodology and
Therapeutic Strategies

EDITED BY

ROBERTO DE FRANCHIS MD

Servizio di Gastroenterologia ed Endoscopia Digestiva,
Istituto di Medicina Interna,
Università degli Studi di Milano,
Milano, Italy

Blackwell
Science

© 1996 by
Blackwell Science Ltd
Editorial Offices:
Osney Mead, Oxford OX2 0EL
25 John Street, London WC1N 2BL
23 Ainslie Place, Edinburgh EH3 6AJ
238 Main Street, Cambridge
  Massachusetts 02142, USA
54 University Street, Carlton
  Victoria 3053, Australia

Other Editorial Offices:
Arnette Blackwell SA
  1, rue de Lille, 75007 Paris
  France

Blackwell Wissenschafts-Verlag GmbH
  Kurfürstendamm 57
  10707 Berlin, Germany

  Feldgasse 13, A-1238 Wien
  Austria

First published 1996

Set by DP Photosetting, Aylesbury, Bucks
Printed and bound in Great Britain
by Hartnolls Ltd, Bodmin, Cornwall

DISTRIBUTORS

Marston Book Services Ltd
PO Box 87
Oxford OX2 0DT
(*Orders:* Tel: 01865 791155
      Fax: 01865 791927
      Telex: 837515)

North America
Blackwell Science, Inc.
238 Main Street
Cambridge, MA 02142
(*Orders:* Tel: 800 215-1000
      617 876-7000
      Fax: 617 492-5263)

Australia
Blackwell Science Pty Ltd
54 University Street
Carlton, Victoria 3053
(*Orders:* Tel: 03 9347 0300
      Fax: 03 9349 3016)

A catalogue record for this title
is available from the British Library

ISBN 0-86542-614-7

Library of Congress
Cataloging-in-Publication Data

Portal hypertension II: proceedings of the
second Baveno international consensus workshop
on definitions, methodology and
therapeutic strategies
edited by Roberto de Franchis.
      p.   cm.
  Includes bibliographical references
  and index.
  ISBN 0-86542-614-7
  1. Portal hypertension—Congresses.
  I. De Franchis, Roberto.
  [DNLM: 1. Hypertension, Portal—congresses.
  2. Gastrointestinal Hemorrhage—congresses.
  WI 720 P8423 1996]
  RC848. P6P662   1996
  616.3′62—dc20
  DNLM/DLC
  for Library of Congress

Contents

Contributors

PAULA ALEXANDRINO MD, *Servicio Medicina II, Hospital Universitario de Santa Maria, Lisbon, Portugal*

GENNARO D'AMICO MD, *Medicina Interna 2, Università di Palermo and Divisione di Medicina, Ospedale 'V. Cervello', Palermo, Italy*

ADELE D'ANTONI MD, *Medicina Interna 2, Università di Palermo and Divisione di Medicina, Ospedale 'V. Cervello', Palermo, Italy*

EMMA ARAGONA MD, *Medicina Interna 2, Università di Palermo and Divisione di Medicina, Ospedale 'V. Cervello', Palermo, Italy*

ALESSANDRO BAISI MD, *Istituto di Chirurgia Generale e Oncologia Chirurgica, Università di Milano, Italy*

GIORGIO BATTAGLIA MD, *Istituto di Chirurgia Generale 2°, Università di Padua, Italy*

ULRIK BECKER MD, *Department of Medical Gastroenterology, Hvidovre University Hospital, Copenhagen, Denmark*

LUIGI BOLONDI MD, *Istituto di Clinica Medica e Gastroenterologia, Università di Bologna, Italy*

JAIME BOSCH MD, *Hepatic Haemodynamic Laboratory, Liver Unit, Hospital Clínic i Provincial, University of Barcelona, Spain*

ANDREW K. BURROUGHS MD, *University Department of Medicine, Royal Free Hospital, London, UK*

PAUL CALÉS MD, *Department of Hepatology and Gastroenterology, Centre Hôspitalier Universitaire, Angers, France*

WOLFGANG FLEIG MD, *First Department of Medicine, Martin Luther University, Halle/Saale, Germany*

ROBERTO DE FRANCHIS MD, *Associate Professor of Medicine, Servizio di Gastroenterologia ed Endoscopia Digestiva, Istituto di Medicina Interna, Università degli Studi di Milano, Italy*

LISA FERAYORNI MD, *Post-graduate Fellow, Veterans Administration Medical Center, Hepatic Hemodynamic Laboratory, West Haven, Connecticut and Yale University School of Medicine, New Haven, Connecticut, USA*

STEFANO GAIANI MD, *Istituto di Clinica Medica e Gastroenterologia, Università di Bologna, Italy*

CHRISTIAN GLUUD MD, *Copenhagen Trial Unit, Institute of Preventive Medicine, Copenhagen Hospital Corporation, Denmark*

NORMAN GRACE MD, *Department of Gastroenterology, Faulkner Hospital, Boston, USA*

ROBERTO J. GROSZMANN MD, *Professor of Medicine, Chief, Digestive Diseases/111J, Veterans Administrative Medical Center, Hepatic Hemodynamic Laboratory, West Haven, Connecticut and Yale University School of Medicine, New Haven, Connecticut, USA*

J. MICHAEL HENDERSON MD, *Department of General Surgery, The Cleveland Clinic Foundation, Cleveland, Ohio, USA*

DIDIER LEBREC MD, *Laboratoire d'Hemodynamique Splanchnique, Unité de Recherches de Physiopathologie Hépatique (INSERM U-24) and Service d'Hépatologie, Hôpital Beaujon, Clichy, France*

ALESSANDRO LIBERATI MD, *The Italian Cochrane Centre, Istituto Mario Negri, Milan, Italy*

GIUSEPPE MALIZIA MD, *Medicina Interna 2, Università di Palermo and Divisione di Medicina, Ospedale 'V. Cervello', Palermo, Italy*

GIORGIO MINOLI MD, *Divisione di Gastroenterologia, Ospedale Valduce, Como, Italy*

ALBERTO MORABITO MD, *Institute of Medical and Biomedical Statistics, University of Milan, Italy*

RICHARD MOREAU MD, *Laboratoire d'Hemodynamique Splanchnique, Unité de Recherches de Physiopathologie Hépatique (INSERM U-24) and Service d'Hépatologie, Hôpital Beaujon, Clichy, France*

LUIGI PAGLIARO MD, *Medicina Interna 2, Università di Palermo and Divisione di Medicina, Ospedale 'V. Cervello', Palermo, Italy*

LINDA PASTA MD, *Medicina Interna 2, Università di Palermo and Divisione di Medicina, Ospedale 'V. Cervello', Palermo, Italy*

ALBERTO PERACCHIA MD, *Istituto di Chirurgia Generale e Oncologia Chirurgica, University of Milan, Italy*

VITTORIO PERI MD, *Medicina Interna 2, Università di Palermo and Divisione di Medicina, Ospedale 'V. Cervello', Palermo, Italy*

FABIO PISCAGLIA MD, *Istituto di Clinica Medica e Gastroenterologia, Università di Bologna, Italy*

JOHN POLIO MD, *Clinical Assistant Professor of Medicine, Veterans Administration Medical Center, Hepatic Hemodynamic Laboratory, West Haven, Connecticut and Yale University School of Medicine, New Haven, Connecticut, USA*

FLAVIA POLITI MD, *Medicina Interna 2, Università di Palermo and Divisione di Medicina, Ospedale 'V. Cervello', Palermo, Italy*

AURELIO PULEO MD, *Medicina Interna 2, Università di Palermo and Divisione di Medicina, Ospedale 'V. Cervello', Palermo, Italy*

JUAN RODÉS MD, *Liver Unit, Department of Medicine, Hospital Clínic i Provincial, University of Barcelona, Spain*

SHIV K. SARIN MD, *Department of Gastroenterology, G.B. Pant Hospital and Maulana Azad Medical College, New Delhi, India*

ROSANNA SIMONETTI MD, *Medicina Interna 2, Università di Palermo and Divisione di Medicina, Ospedale 'V. Cervello', Palermo, Italy*

SEBASTIANO SIRINGO MD, *Istituto di Clinica Medica e Gastroenterologia, Università di Bologna, Italy*

GIUSEPPE SPATOLIATORE MD, *Medicina Interna 2, Università di Palermo and Divisione di Medicina, Ospedale 'V. Cervello', Palermo, Italy*

FABIO TINÉ MD, *Medicina Interna 2, Università di Palermo and Divisione di Medicina, Ospedale 'V. Cervello', Palermo, Italy*

GIOVANNI VIZZINI MD, *Medicina Interna 2, Università di Palermo and Divisione di Medicina, Ospedale 'V. Cervello', Palermo, Italy*

DAVID WESTABY MA FRCP, *The Department of Gastroenterology, Chelsea and Westminster Hospital, London, UK*

SIMON G.J. WILLIAMS MA MRCP, *The Department of Gastroenterology, Chelsea and Westminster Hospital, London, UK*

GIANNI ZIRONI MD, *Istituto di Clinica Medica e Gastroenterologia, Università di Bologna, Italy*

PARTICIPANTS

Italy: G. Battaglia, L. Bolondi, L. Cestari, R. de Franchis, A. Gatta, G. Gerunda, A. Liberati, A. Maffei Faccioli, C. Merkel, G. Minoli, A. Morabito, L. Pagliaro, A. Peracchia, M. Primignani, O. Riggio, P. Rossi, C. Sabbà, P. Spina, F. Tiné, V. Ziparo
Belgium: F. Nevens
Canada: N. Marcon, G. Pomier-Layrargues
Denmark: U. Becker, F. Bendtsen, C. Gluud
France: P. Cales, D. Lebrec, J.P. Vinel
Germany: K. Binmöller, W. Fleig, G. Richter, M. Rössle, T. Sauerbruch
India: S.K. Sarin
The Netherlands: H. van Buuren
Portugal: P. Alexandrino
Spain: J. Bosch, J. Rodés
Sweden: C. Søderlund
UK: A.K. Burroughs, D. Westaby
USA: N. Grace, R. Groszmann, J.M. Henderson, G. van Stiegmann

Preface

The value of diagnostic tools and the precise role of the available therapeutic modalities in the management of patients with portal hypertension and variceal bleeding has always been difficult to assess. Three main reasons account for this: first, variceal bleeding is a medical emergency, which makes the evaluation of diagnostic methods and the design and conduct of good trials difficult. Second, treatment of bleeding does not treat cirrhosis itself, and therefore the outcome of trials aimed at treating the acute haemorrhage or at preventing first bleeding or rebleeding is heavily influenced by the severity of the underlying liver disease. Third, interpreting the results of trials and placing them in the context of previous work is often very difficult because trials differ widely, both in methodological quality and in the way of reporting information about patients and methods. Awareness of these difficulties led to the organization of two international workshops which were held in Groningen, The Netherlands, in 1986, thanks to the efforts of Andrew Burroughs, and in Baveno, Italy, in 1990, under the sponsorship of the New Italian Endoscopic Club, with the aim of reaching consensus of the definition of some key events related to variceal bleeding and of producing guidelines for the conduct of future studies in this field. Although both meetings made valuable attempts to achieve a better mutual understanding and produced consensus definitions on some important points, a great deal of work remained to be done. In addition, since the Baveno 1990 meeting, a great number of studies have expanded our knowledge on the pathophysiology, diagnosis and treatment of portal hypertension. Moreover, new diagnostic and therapeutic tools have been introduced, which might lead to profound changes in the management of this condition. Thus, my colleagues in the New Italian Endoscopic Club and I considered that the time had come to evaluate the impact of this new knowledge and of these new tools on the diagnostic and therapeutic strategies that we follow in managing patients with portal hypertension. Therefore, with the help and encouragement of a group of friends from 13 countries, many of whom had taken part in the first Baveno workshop, we organized a Baveno II workshop on April 27–28,

1995. The aim of Baveno II was twofold: first, to review and put into perspective the advances in our understanding of portal hypertension, as well as the role of the new diagnostic and therapeutic techniques that have been introduced during the past 5 years. Second, to continue the effort, which had begun in Groningen and had been continued in Baveno I, of producing updated definitions and guidelines aimed at improving the quality of our future studies. We were very fortunate in being able to bring to this workshop some of the experts responsible for most of the major achievements of the last 5 years in this field.

The structure of the Baveno II workshop included nine sessions and four lectures. The first session was devoted to reviewing the points on which a consensus had been reached at Baveno I. In the second session, the points on which there was disagreement at Baveno I were addressed, and an effort was made to bring about a consensus on them. In each of the other seven sessions, the Chairman reviewed and discussed with the panellists an important topic related to the diagnosis or the treatment of portal hypertension. At the end of each session, the Chairman proposed a series of statements that were discussed with the panellists and the other experts on the floor, with the aim of reaching a consensus among the experts on crucial diagnostic, therapeutic and methodological issues. The four lectures were critical evaluations of different aspects of portal hypertension given by four authorities in the field: they addressed the evolution of knowledge on the pathophysiology of portal hypertension, the history of surgery, the possible future evolution of medical therapy, and the process of transferring the experience of trials into clinical practice. These proceedings follow closely the structure of the workshop. The order of sessions and lectures is exactly the same, and the consensus statements that were agreed upon at the end of each session are reported at the end of the pertinent chapters.

We are grateful to all the friends who accepted to give the lectures and to serve as chairmen and panellists of the sessions, and who helped us by working hard in the preparation of the workshop and of the chapters. We also wish to thank Sandra Covre and her staff of Area Congressi, who managed brilliantly the organization of the workshop, Paolo Arcidiacono, Luca de Franchis and Gimmy Meucci who skilfully operated the computer–videoprojector systems during the consensus phase of each session. In addition, we are most grateful to Ferring AB who made the publication of this book possible through a generous grant, to Per J. Wilhelmson for his encouragement and cooperation in this project, and to Blackwell Science for the timely and excellent production of this volume.

ROBERTO DE FRANCHIS
on behalf of the New Italian Endoscopic Club

Where Were We?

A summary of the issues where consensus
was reached at Baveno I

Luigi Pagliaro (Chairman) and Roberto de Franchis

INTRODUCTION

In 1990 the New Italian Endoscopic Club (NIEC) organized an International
Consensus Workshop on definitions, methodology and therapeutic strategies
in portal hypertension, which was held at Baveno, Italy on April 5 and 6,
1990 (Baveno I) [1]. The workshop was aimed at establishing a uniform
nomenclature and consensus definitions concerning several aspects of portal
hypertension and variceal bleeding. These definitions were intended as
workable tools which were to be used in designing and carrying out future
trials.

At Baveno I, the following issues were addressed: (i) endoscopic aspects of
portal hypertension and variceal bleeding; (ii) diagnosis of variceal bleeding
and of clinically significant bleeding; (iii) time events in the variceal bleeding
episode; (iv) patients classification – how and when; (v) prognostic factors
for first and further bleeding or survival; (vi) imaging techniques in portal
hypertension; (vii) value of variceal pressure measurements; (viii) definition
of therapeutic strategies; and (ix) methodological requirements of future
trials.

In the present chapter, we report the issues on which consensus was
reached at Baveno I.

Baveno I Consensus Statements

ENDOSCOPIC ASPECTS OF PORTAL HYPERTENSION AND VARICEAL BLEEDING – CONSENSUS

I Oesophageal varices

1   Only one classification should be used in all circumstances, i.e. in daily
practice or for clinical research.

1

2   The classification should be as simple as possible, i.e. in two grades, large and small.

3   Among other parameters used in current classifications (colour, form, location, appearance of the surface, number of chords) only the presence or absence of red signs on varices seems relevant.

II Gastric varices

1   The location of gastric varices is important and any description should distinguish between:

    (a) varices of the cardia; and

    (b) varices of the fornix (true gastric varices).

2   Assessment of the size of gastric varices is difficult.

3   Assessment of the location of the bleeding point on a gastric varix is extremely difficult, with a high rate of error if endoscopy is performed in the haemorrhagic period.

III Portal-hypertension-related gastropathy

As of 1990, hypertensive gastropathy should be classified only as present or absent.

DIAGNOSIS OF VARICEAL BLEEDING AND DEFINITION OF CLINICALLY SIGNIFICANT BLEEDING – CONSENSUS

I Diagnosis of variceal bleeding

1   Endoscopy should be done as soon as possible.

2   The timing of endoscopy with respect to bleeding must be reported in studies for further evaluation.

3   Active bleeding: diagnosis certain.

4   Signs of recent bleeding:

    (a) 'white nipple' – certain;

    (b) if clot – wash!

5   Varices without other sources: diagnosis certain when blood is present in stomach and/or if endoscopy is made within 24 hours.

II Significance of active bleeding at endoscopy

No consensus could be reached on this point.

III Definition of bleeding and of clinically significant bleeding

1   Bleeding: occurrence of haematemesis and/or melaena or gastric aspirate containing blood.
2   Clinically significant bleeding: no consensus could be reached on this point.

TIME EVENTS IN THE VARICEAL BLEEDING EPISODE – CONSENSUS

I Time zero

The time of admission to the first hospital the patient is taken to is time zero.

II Definition of duration of acute bleeding episode and factors used to assess failure to control bleeding

No consensus could be reached on this point.

III Severity of rebleeding; IV Rebleeding index; V Source of rebleeding

No consensus could be reached on these points.

VI Definition of death related to variceal bleeding and mode of death

Any death within 6 weeks of time zero would be a death related to bleeding, regardless of the mode of death. Thirty-day mortality (a surgical convention) and deaths during admission should also be reported. The latter is solely descriptive. The starting point for all three time intervals is time zero. The immediately precipitating causes of death should be described, and represent the mode of death.

PATIENT CLASSIFICATION, HOW AND WHEN – CONSENSUS

1   The Child–Pugh classification is still the most useful and practical tool to classify patients. It should be calculated from data collected at randomization.
2   Aetiology should be stated for patients entered into trials. The severity of cirrhosis is probably more important for prognosis. Histological confirmation is not an absolute requirement.
3   The occurrence of concomitant renal insufficiency, cardiopulmonary

changes, nutritional impairment and sepsis may all have a major impact on outcome, and should be addressed in defining patient populations in randomized trials. As a minimum recommendation, serum creatinine and/or blood urea nitrogen should be included in defining study groups.

4   Portal pressure measurements and/or quantitative data (Galactose elimination capacity (GEC), indocyanine green (ICG), caffeine) can be selectively assessed in trials for explanatory purposes.

5   Differentiate between: (i) acute studies and chronic studies – complex diagnostic work-up is not feasible in the acute situation; (ii) clinical studies and scientific studies, in which more sophisticated measurements are justified.

PROGNOSTIC FACTORS FOR FIRST AND FURTHER BLEEDING – CONSENSUS

I Risk factors for first bleeding

1   It is important to assess the risk of first bleeding.

2   Simple endoscopic criteria such as variceal size and red signs, possibly in combination with the Child–Pugh score as in the NIEC index should be used to assess the risk of first bleeding.

3   The evaluation should be repeated at yearly intervals.

4   Prospective information on the risk of first bleeding available today is insufficient and should be extended by further studies, including possibly additional (haemodynamic?) parameters.

II Risk factors for early bleeding and death

No consensus could be reached on these points.

III Risk factors for late rebleeding and death

No consensus could be reached on these points.

IMAGING TECHNIQUES IN PORTAL HYPERTENSION – CONSENSUS

1   As of 1990, angiography is still the 'gold standard' of all imaging techniques available for the study of portal hypertensive patients, especially in the preoperative and postoperative stages. This may change as experience accumulates with newer techniques.

2   Echography is a good screening procedure, but when the results are in doubt it should be complemented by angiography.

3   With the exception of angiography for surgical patients, the usefulness of imaging techniques in the follow-up of portal hypertensive patients has not been demonstrated. This is an area where the potential usefulness of the echo–Doppler technique should be explored.

4   The potential of newer techniques such as nuclear magnetic resonance and endoscopic ultrasonography should be explored further.

VALUE OF VARICEAL PRESSURE MEASUREMENTS – CONSENSUS

1   Direct puncture of the variceal wall to measure variceal pressure is not a routine procedure. The risks are not well defined. Moreover, interpretation of the results may be difficult, and should be done carefully.

2   Direct puncture of the variceal wall may be justified for investigational purposes only. Preferably, sclerotherapy should be scheduled immediately after the procedure.

3   The existing experience on the use of indirect methods (pressure-sensitive capsules or balloons) is still too limited to allow any conclusion.

DEFINING THERAPEUTIC STRATEGIES – CONSENSUS

I Prevention of first bleeding

1   Patients with small varices should not receive prophylaxis of first variceal haemorrhage, except in trials.

2   All patients with high variceal bleeding risk should receive prophylaxis of first variceal bleeding. At present, beta-blockers are the best candidate drugs.

3   (i) Endoscopic criteria have the highest value in defining the risk of bleeding; (ii) reliable standardization of these criteria is still lacking; and (iii) further criteria may be important (liver function, aetiology of cirrhosis).

II Treatment of acute variceal bleeding

1   Acute oesophageal variceal bleeding.
   (a) First-choice therapy – consensus could be achieved only on the following statement: in every centre a treatment strategy should be defined, with several steps to control the bleeding episode, not only for 24 hours, but for a few days (e.g. 5), with strictly defined criteria for failure of every treatment option used.

2   Acute bleeding from gastric varices:
   (a) vasoactive drugs/tamponade (Linton tube);
   (b) laparotomy (decompressive shunts).

III Prevention of recurrent bleeding

1 First-choice therapy to prevent rebleeding: no consensus could be reached on this point. However, there was consensus that 'no treatment' is not justified: endoscopic sclerotherapy, beta-blockers or surgery can be used. The patient's condition must be taken into account when making the choice (i.e. Child C patients should not be treated by shunt surgery).
2 If the first choice of treatment failed: endoscopic sclerotherapy, beta-blockers, surgical shunt and liver transplantation can all be used.
3 First choice for prevention of gastric variceal rebleeding: beta-blockers. Surgery and endoscopic sclerotherapy can, however, be used.

METHODOLOGICAL REQUIREMENTS OF FUTURE TRIALS – CONSENSUS

I Major outcome measures

1 Prevention of first bleeding:
  (a) first variceal bleeding;
  (b) death before variceal bleeding;
  (c) course, including death, after variceal bleeding.
2 Treatment of acute bleeding:
  (a) control of bleeding;
  (b) death within 42 days after bleeding.
3 Prevention of rebleeding:
  (a) variceal rebleeding;
  (b) death before variceal rebleeding;
  (c) course, including death, after variceal rebleeding.

II Subsidiary outcome measures

1 Clinical course:
  (a) causes of death, especially bleeding;
  (b) liver function (encephalopathy);
  (c) upper gastrointestinal bleeding from non-variceal sources.
2 Cost of treatment:
  (a) side effects and complications;
  (b) time in hospital and intensive care unit.
3 Additional treatment:
  (a) transfusion;
  (b) ancillary treatment.
4 Overall results:

(a) quality of life;
(b) cost–benefit.
5 Paraclinical aspects as surrogates of potential clinical effects:
(a) variceal size;
(b) haemodynamics.

III Sample size calculation

1 Essential part of the planning of trials expected to produce conclusive results on major end-points.
2 It should be included in the final report of any trial.

IV Double blindness

1 Useful to avoid biased assessment of outcomes in which there is a subjective component, either for the physician or for the patient.
2 Useful to avoid biased approaches to patients, by physicians, staff, relatives and patients themselves, with possible influence on the clinical course.
3 Necessary for the distinction between specific biological effects and general effects of administration of the treatment.
4 Should be used whenever possible.

V Randomization

1 Use randomization for allocation of treatments to be compared.
2 Randomization must be closed, i.e. the treatment must not be known before the decision to include the patient is made.

VI Stratification in randomization

1 Always by centre in multicentre trials.
2 By one or two well-defined and easily accessible variables of great prognostic significance in trials including less than 100 patients.

VII Exclusion before randomization

1 Patients evaluated and fulfilling the entry criteria but not randomized must be reported.

VIII Intention to treat analysis

1   Include all randomized patients with outcomes recorded at any time until closure of the trial in the analysis.

2   An analysis as 'per treatment received' should be performed which only excludes patients who actually did not start treatment. This analysis should include entry characteristics to establish balance.

IX Exclusions after randomization

1   Patients withdrawn from the trial or lost to follow-up need to be described and analysed.

X Competing end-points

1   Should be taken into account in the analysis and interpretation of the results.

XI Stratification in analysis

1   Several variables may be taken into account in multivariate analysis, but it is advisable to decide which variables in the planning of the trial.

2   The variables used for stratification before randomization should be included.

XII Management of the patients in the control group

1   Prevention of first bleeding: no consensus was reached on whether no treatment or placebo is justified.

2   Treatment of acute bleeding: some accepted form of treatment must be given.

3   Prevention of rebleeding: no treatment is not justified – sclerotherapy, beta-blockers or surgery must be used.

META-ANALYSIS, GOOD NEWS AND BAD NEWS – CONSENSUS

1   When there is clear heterogeneity across the results of randomized controlled trials (RCTs), or they are clearly different for clinical characteristics, pooling will result in a loss of information rather than in a gain. In the absence of heterogeneity, meta-analysis is useful for obtaining cumulative information from a multitude of RCTs.

2   Meta-analysis must improve in methodology: extensive search for trials, preliminary analysis of clinical characteristics, sound criteria for omitting or including trials, statistical and graphic evaluation of heterogeneity, and balanced conclusions from pooled estimates are all relevant issues.

3   There is a reciprocal relationship between meta-analysis and trials. Good trials are needed for a reliable meta-analysis, and meta-analysis can result in new ideas and better-designed RCTs. Improving both sides of this relationship should be our aim in the future.

REFERENCE

1 de Franchis R, Pascal JP, Ancona E *et al*. Definitions, methodology and therapeutic strategies in portal hypertension. A consensus development workshop. *J Hepatol* 1992; **15**: 256–261.

'Sore Points'

A review of the points where there was disagreement at Baveno I, and an attempt to reach consensus

Andrew K. Burroughs (Chairman), Paula Alexandrino, Paul Calés, Wolfgang Fleig, Norman Grace, Giorgio Minoli and Sebastiano Siringo

INTRODUCTION

There were several areas in which consensus could not be reached at Baveno I [1]. For example, there was no consensus on definitions for clinically significant bleeding, failure to control acute bleeding, duration of the acute bleeding episode, rebleeding episodes (both in terms of severity and sources) or a rebleeding index. There was also no agreement on algorithms for treatment of variceal bleeding and prevention of bleeding, nor about the finding of active bleeding at endoscopy and how to classify patients.

As a background for this session, a questionnaire covering the above unresolved issues was sent to all the panellists from different centres in all the sessions in Baveno II. There were 37 centres, and there was a response from 30 (81%). This group was represented by 21 physicians (internists), eight surgeons and one radiologist. The countries represented were as follows: Italy ($n = 10$), Germany ($n = 5$), USA ($n = 2$), France ($n = 2$), UK ($n = 2$), Denmark ($n = 2$), Canada ($n = 2$), Sweden ($n = 1$), Netherlands ($n = 1$) and Belgium ($n = 1$). The results of the questionnaire formed the basis of discussion with the audience and the consensus statements.

ACTIVE BLEEDING AT ENDOSCOPY

Active bleeding at endoscopy was felt to be of prognostic significance for short-term mortality (yes = 15, no = 8, do not know = 7) and for early rebleeding (yes = 15, no = 9, do not know = 6). For most experts, active bleeding at endoscopy changed the therapeutic approach (yes = 21, no = 9). Despite this apparent majority view it was clear from the discussion that there was not a consensus to come to an agreement. In fact, there are very few studies on the prognostic significance of active bleeding seen endoscopically in variceal bleeding [2]. Moreover, studies in many cases are complicated by the frequent use of vasoactive drugs before the diagnostic endoscopy. In addition there is often no differentiation between oozing and spurting and the influence of the timing of endoscopy.

Consensus statement for active bleeding

Active bleeding is an important clinical descriptor for which it is not clear if it has prognostic significance. The following should be described in clinical studies and trials: oozing or spurting, timing of endoscopy (from time zero) and treatment before endoscopy. Studies in acute variceal bleeding should evaluate the importance of active bleeding.

Most centres believed it to be useful to stage variceal size and document the presence of red signs at the initial diagnostic endoscopy (yes = 21, no = 7, do not know = 2), so that size of varices should also be evaluated prognostically for the short term.

CLINICALLY SIGNIFICANT BLEEDING

Most centres felt it was necessary to define clinically significant bleeding (yes = 20, no = 9, do not know = 1). The four variables considered most useful to define this were as follows: blood pressure (yes = 22, no = 4, do not know = 4), pulse (yes = 19, no = 7, do not know = 4), transfusion of blood (yes = 18, no = 8, do not know = 4), haematocrit (Hct) or haemoglobin (Hb) (yes = 17, no = 9, do not know = 4).

The cut-off points used were systolic blood pressure < 100 mmHg (n= 14), < 80 mmHg (n = 3), < 95 mmHg (n = 1); pulse > 100 (n = 14), > 110 (n = 2), > 120 (n = 1); units transfused, 2 units (n = 9), 4 units (n = 4), 1 unit (n = 3); and haemoglobin < 8 g/dl (n = 6); > 2 g/dl drop (n = 4), < 9 g/dl (n = 2).

Despite the need to define clinically significant bleeding, most centres – but not all – counted any bleeding episode (as defined in Baveno I) regardless of its severity, as bleeding (yes = 24, no = 4, do not know = 2).

Consensus definition on clinically significant bleeding

A transfusion requirement of 2 units of blood or more within 24 hours of time zero, together with a systolic blood pressure < 100 mmHg or a postural change of < 20 mmHg and/or pulse rate < 100/min, at time zero.

In addition it was agreed that the following were to be recorded: admission Hct or Hb and the lowest values within 24 hours and also beta-blocker treatment before bleeding as this may affect blood pressure and pulse.

The variables considered the most important in defining clinically significant bleeding have all been shown to be associated with identifying a poor prognosis for upper gastrointestinal bleeding in general [3–6].

FAILURE TO CONTROL ACUTE BLEEDING

Most centres defined this in their own centres (yes = 26, no = 2, do not know = 2). The reasons for defining failure were: so as to add or change therapy (yes = 26, do not know = 3); to increase clinical monitoring (yes = 16, no = 12, do not know = 2); and for clinical trial purposes (yes = 16, no = 11, do not know = 3). It was clear that there was a clinical reason to define this as 26 responded no, and four do not know when asked if they used their definition for no clinical reasons, but just for description.

The most important variables used to define failure were: recurrent haematemesis (yes = 21, no = 6, do not know = 3), systolic blood pressure (yes = 18, no = 8, do not know = 4), recurrence of melaena (yes = 18, no = 8, do not know = 4), transfusion of blood (yes = 16, no = 10, do not know = 4) and pulse (yes = 16, no = 11, do not know = 3).

The limits set were as follows for blood pressure: < 100 mmHg ($n = 8$), < 90 mmHg ($n = 4$), < 80 mmHg ($n = 2$), no limits set ($n = 4$). For pulse they were > 100/min ($n = 10$), > 120/min ($n = 3$), no limits ($n = 3$).

For transfusion there was a separation in the need for blood within 6 hours and the amount transfused within 24 hours. Within 6 hours the amounts set as limits were as follows: 6 units ($n = 4$), 5 units ($n = 1$), 4 units ($n = 1$), 3 units ($n = 1$), 2 units ($n = 3$). For the limits within 24 hours the limits set were as follows: 6 units ($n = 1$), 4 units ($n = 1$), 3 units ($n = 2$), 2 units ($n = 2$).

Only four centres considered transfusion of blood and colloid as the important criteria, whereas 16 centres used transfused blood alone.

The consensus definition of failure to control bleeding was divided into two time frames

1   Failure to control acute variceal bleeding within 6 hours is defined as any of the following three factors: (a) transfusion of 4 units of blood or more; (b) inability to achieve an increase in systolic blood pressure by a 20 mmHg or to 70 mmHg or more; (c) and/or pulse reduction to less than 100/min or a reduction of 10/min from baseline pulse rate. Use of vasoactive drugs should be taken into account and their use recorded.
2   Failure to control acute variceal bleeding after 6 hours is defined as any of the following 4 factors: (a) the occurrence of haematemesis; (b) reduction in blood pressure ⩾ 20 mmHg from the 6-hour point; (c) and/or

increase in pulse rate $\geqslant$ 20/min from the 6-hour point on two consecutive readings an hour apart; (d) transfusion of 2 units of blood or more (over and above the previous transfusion) required to increase the Hct $\geqslant$ 27% or Hb $\geqslant$ 9 g/dl.

TIME FRAME FOR THE ACUTE VARICEAL BLEEDING EPISODE

Most centres used a time frame to encompass the acute variceal bleeding episode. This was because it should be separated from the first rebleeding episode (particularly in clinical trials), and because there is a distinction between therapy for acute bleeding and that used to prevent rebleeding.

An important consideration not taken into account by most respondents was the fact that most endoscopic therapy is only re-administered at least 3 and up to 7 days after the emergency endoscopic therapy, and beta-blockers are not introduced until after at least 2, more often 3 days of haemodynamic stability. Thus, there appears to be a gap between the time frame encompassing an acute bleeding episode and the time point for the start of prevention of rebleeding. The centres responded as follows regarding this time frame: 24 hours ($n = 13$), 12 hours ($n = 6$), 6 hours ($n = 3$), 2 days ($n = 3$), 5 days ($n = 3$), not specified ($n = 2$). In addition, a further question was asked regarding when it was considered that rebleeding occurred in relation to an interval of stability after an admission with acute bleeding. This interval was > 24 hours ($n = 14$), > 12 hours ($n = 8$), > 5 days ($n = 2$), > 48 hours ($n = 1$), 76 hours ($n = 1$), > 1 hour ($n = 1$) and not specified ($n = 3$).

Thus, from the answers to these two questions the period encompassing the acute bleeding episode was 48 hours for most centres, as most favoured a 24-hour period encompassing 'bleeding' and 24 hours of stability.

Consensus definition for the time frame for acute bleeding

The acute bleeding episode is represented by an interval of 48 hours from time zero with no evidence of clinically significant bleeding between 24 and 48 hours. Evidence of any bleeding after 48 hours is the first rebleeding episode.

REBLEEDING: DEFINITIONS

The same defined criteria as for the initial bleeding were used by 24 respondents, with three using different criteria and three said they did not know. However, in evaluating rebleeds, 15 of 30 respondents only counted a rebleed if it was clinically significant, with 13 counting any rebleeding regardless of severity as a rebleeding episode and two replies were 'do not know'.

Consensus definition for rebleeding

The occurrence of new haematemesis or new melaena after a period of 24 hours or more from the 24 hours point of stable vital signs and Hct/Hb following an episode of acute bleeding. Clinically significant rebleeds should be evaluated as a separate end point and all rebleeding regardless of severity should be counted in evaluating rebleeding.

There was also initial disagreement on the sources of rebleeding to be evaluated. Only 13 considered all rebleeds as the end point, and 13 excluded peptic ulceration bleeds. A majority of 26 considered only oesophageal variceal bleeds as evaluable end-points. They excluded bleeds due to peptic ulceration, gastric mucosal lesions and gastric varices. These varying responses were a surplus as it was not appreciated that there was such disagreement on an apparently clear-cut end-point.

The consensus was to describe all rebleeding events and to use subgroup analyses for the individual sources. Sources said to be unknown should be evaluated with portal hypertensive bleeds.

Finally a rebleeding index was agreed upon in order to evaluate: (i) patients with more than one rebleed; (ii) patients who never rebled; (iii) the interval without rebleeding; and (iv) to give a measure of distribution. The rebleeding index is:

$$\frac{\text{episodes of rebleeding} + 1}{\text{months of follow up per patient}}$$

This fulfils all the considerations above.

CLASSIFICATION OF PATIENTS

There was general agreement that Child's classification remains the most useful tool to classify patients. The Child–Pugh classification is probably preferable to the Child–Turcotte because prothrombin time is easier to quantitate than nutritional status. However, there are no data that either classification is otherwise preferable. At least 27 of 30 respondents used each variable to classify patients, including 20 who always used prothrombin time. Most importantly, determination of the Child's status should be based upon a point system with the total numerical score determining the patient's status and not the single worst characteristic [7]. The Pugh scoring system has 5 or 6 points for grade A, 7, 8 or 9 for grade B, and 10–15 for grade C. The score should be assessed at time zero and if used at other time points this should be described.

Over half the respondents ($n = 7$) felt that the creatinine was useful as an indicator of renal insufficiency and had prognostic significance. Recording of variceal size and endoscopic red colour signs were useful for prediction of first variceal haemorrhage but are of descriptive value only for rebleeding as all these patients require therapy [8,9]. There was consensus that quantitative liver function tests, while of potential interest, had not been demonstrated to give additional information of a prognostic nature and, therefore, were not necessary for classification of patients.

Although there was no complete agreement about the use of portal haemodynamic measurements for classification of patients, there are increasing data that suggest that measurements of the hepatic venous pressure gradient have prognostic significance for survival but not for variceal bleeding [10–12]. Future studies should evaluate this. Doppler ultrasonography is a potentially very useful non-invasive means of assessing portal haemodynamics but, at present, has problems with equipment and observer variability and is observer-dependent [7].

TREATMENT ALGORITHMS

Algorithm for acute variceal bleeding

Only 15 out of 30 gave some information about the algorithm used in their unit and the answers were different and difficult to summarize and evaluate. Most of the experts believe that resuscitation measures and vasoactive drugs (vasopressin, somatostatin, Octreotide) are the first step (12 of 15) and that endoscopic treatment has to be performed as soon as possible (15 of 15).

Treatment for acute bleeding from gastric varices

Vasoactive drugs ($n = 21$), transjugular intrahepatic portosystemic shunt (TIPS) ($n = 20$), decompressive shunts ($n = 16$) and adhesive injections ($n = 15$) were the most popular treatments: devascularization ($n = 10$) and sclerotherapy ($n = 9$) with sclerosants or thrombotic agents are used only by a minority. Very few (four out of 14) used band ligation.

Algorithm for acute gastric variceal bleeding

The answers were 24 (out of 30) and, as was the case of the oesophageal varices algorithm, it was difficult to summarize. Vasoactive drugs and resuscitation measures ($n = 19$) are the first step, followed by TIPS or decompressive shunt ($n = 19$), bucrylate ($n = 11$), and sclerotherapy ($n = 8$) as the second step.

Treatment for rebleeding

The first-choice treatment for rebleeding was usually sclerotherapy alone ($n = 17$) or associated with banding ($n = 2$) or beta-blockers ($n = 2$). Beta-blockers alone are rarely used ($n = 4$), which was surprising considering the evidence of efficacy in trials vs. sclerotherapy. In case of contraindications for the first-choice treatment, the options were many and without any agreement. In case of failure of the first-choice treatment, TIPS was the preferred treatment by 10 out of 21 respondents. *There was no consensus on the definitions of failure of treatment for rebleeding and for failure to prevent rebleeding.* As for the disagreement about the definition of rebleeding, this was somewhat surprising. As an example, failure of treatment to prevent rebleeding was defined as: one rebleed ($n = 6$), including three after eradications, two rebleeds ($n = 6$), and more than three clinically significant rebleeds ($n = 3$). The time intervals in which these rebleeds were evaluated were either within 6 or 12 months of follow-up.

> The consensus was that failure to prevent rebleeding should be precisely defined according to severity, number and sources of rebleeding. It is hoped that this will be a situation for which there will be consensus in the future.

SUMMARY

The purpose of these consensus definitions is to use them in clinical trials and studies of variceal bleeding. This does not mean that authors cannot use their own definitions, but they should use and evaluate them in parallel with these Baveno II consensus definitions. This should bring about some standardization and increased ease of interpretation among different studies. More importantly, if there are common end-points, meta-analyses will be based on trials evaluating the same end-points which is the *sine qua non* of this methodology. We as authors make a joint appeal to report future studies using these definitions as part of the evaluation. Change or refinement can then take place to ensure that the consensus definitions do have clinical relevance and are easily applied in practice.

REFERENCES

1 de Franchis R, Pascal JP, Ancona E *et al.* Definitions, methodology and therapeutic strategies on portal hypertension. *J Hepatol* 1992; **15**: 256–261.
2 Cardin F, Gori G, McCormick PA, Burroughs AK. A predictive model for very early rebleeding from varices (abstract). *Gut* 1990; **31**: A1204.
3 Burroughs AK, Siringo S, McCormick PA. Design of studies to modify the natural history. In Bosch J, Rodes J (eds), *Recent Advances in the Pathophysiology and Therapy of Portal Hypertension.* Serono Symposia Review No. 22. Ares Serono Symposia, Rome, 1989: 207–218.
4 Silverstein FE, Gilbert DA, Tedesco FJ, Buenger NK, Persing J. The national ASCE survey on upper gastrointestinal bleeding. II clinical prognostic factors. *Gastrointest Endosc* 1981; **27**: 80–93.
5 Clason AE, Maclead DAD, Elton RE. Clinical factors in the prediction of further haemorrhage or mortality in acute gastrointestinal haemorrhage. *Br J Surg* 1986; **73**: 985–987.
6 De Dombal FT, Clark JR, Clamp SE, Malizia G, Kotwal MR, Morgan AG. Prognostic factors in upper GI bleeding. *Endoscopy* 1986; **18** (Suppl. 2): 6–10.
7 Conn HO. A peek at Child–Turcotte classification. *Hepatology* 1981; **1**: 673–676.
8 The North Italian Endoscopic Club for the Study and treatment of oesophageal varices. Prediction of the variceal haemorrhage in patients with cirrhosis of the liver and oesophageal varices: a prospective multicenter study. *N Engl J Med* 1988; **319**: 983–989.
9 Rigo GP, Merighi A, Chalin NJ *et al.* A prospective study of the ability of three endoscopic classifications to predict haemorrhage from oesophageal varices. *Gastrointest Endosc* 1992; **39**: 425–429.
10 Merkel C, Bolognesi M, Bellon S *et al.* Prognostic usefulness of hepatic vein catheterization in patients with cirrhosis and oesophageal varices. *Gastroenterology* 1991; **102**: 973–979.
11 Vinel JP, Cassigneul J, Levade M, Voigt JJ, Pascal JP. Assessment of short-term prognosis after variceal bleeding in patients with alcoholic cirrhosis by yearly measurements of portohepatic gradient. *Hepatology* 1986; **6**: 116–117.
12 Barrett G, Bosch J, Garcia-Tsao G *et al.* Hepatic venous pressure gradient as a predictor of survival in patients with cirrhosis. *Hepatology* 1990; **21**: 850(A).
13 Sabba C, Merkel C, Zoli M *et al.* Inter-observer and inter-equipment variability of echo doppler examination of the portal vein: effect of a cooperative training programme. *Hepatology* 1995; **21**: 428–433.

The Evolution of Knowledge on the Pathophysiology of Portal Hypertension

Juan Rodés

INTRODUCTION

Portal hypertension is a common complication of a great variety of both acute and chronic liver diseases. It is characterized by an increase in portal venous pressure which stimulates the development of portosystemic collaterals and therefore the passage of part of the portal blood to the systemic circulation producing humoral and haemodynamic alterations.

Hepatic cirrhosis is the most frequent cause of portal hypertension. Initially the pathophysiology of portal hypertension in cirrhosis was considered 70 years ago as a consequence of an increased resistance to portal blood flow induced by hepatic sclerosis or even by a compression of the hepatic nodules to hepatic sinusoids [1,2]. At present, however, it seems that, in addition to this mechanical mechanism, there are neurohumoral factors that may play a central role in the development of this syndrome [3]. In patients with cirrhosis, increased resistance to blood flow is located in the hepatic sinusoids [4].

SINUSOIDS

The hepatic sinusoids are structurally unique among microvessels since they do not have a basement membrane. They are lined by four main types of cells: endothelial cells, Kupffer cells, pit cells and fat-storing cells (Ito cells)[5]. The endothelial cells are, by far, the main component of the sinusoidal wall. Although Kupffer cells also contribute to the sinusoidal wall, they are often located in the sinusoidal lumen. The most important function of Kupffer cells is to phagocytize many substances such as denaturated albumin, bacteria and immune complexes. Pit cells are large granular lymphocytes and they are in contact with Kupffer or endothelial cells. These cells may play a role in defence against tumoural cells and viruses. Ito cells are found in the space of Disse. They contain lipids including vitamin A. These cells belong to the fibromyoblast family [6].

The endothelial cells form a very porous sinusoidal wall with large apertures (fenestrated endothelial barrier), ranging from 100 to 500 nm in radius. This facilitates exchange between incoming blood and hepatocytes through the space of Disse, as well as immunological defence mechanisms [6]. Hepatic sinusoidal circulation is initiated undirectionally in zone 1 (periportal) to zone 3 (perivenular) of the Rappaport's acinus. Sinusoidal microcirculation is variable in the rat. This variability is due to the presence of inlet, sinusoidal and outlet sphincters. These sphincters have not yet been described in humans [5].

PATHOPHYSIOLOGY OF PORTAL HYPERTENSION

As in any vascular system, the pressure gradient along the portal venous system is the result of the product of portal blood flow and vascular resistance. Therefore this relationship, according to Ohm's law, is defined by the equation:

$$P = Q \times R$$

in which P is the portal pressure gradient Q is the blood flow and R is the vascular resistance of the portal venous system. As a consequence of this relationship, portal pressure may increase when there is an increase in vascular resistance and/or high portal blood flow.

Increased vascular resistance

The initial event in the pathophysiology of portal hypertension is the increased vascular resistance to portal flow at any site of the portal venous system. As indicated in the introduction, portal hypertension in cirrhosis has been related to the development of hepatic fibrosis, scarring and nodule formation [3]. More recently, it has been shown that hepatic necrosis and portal inflammation also cause an increase in vascular resistance. These data suggest that the mechanical phenomena responsible for portal hypertension in cirrhosis or acute hepatitis may be variable and the predominance of each depends on the type and the stage of the hepatic disease [7].

The cause of an increased intrasinusoidal pressure in patients with cirrhosis regardless of aetiology remains a matter of debate. It is considered that a loss of endothelial fenestrations, sinusoidal narrowing and changes in the distensibility of sinusoids, may produce a mechanical obstruction to blood flow [8,9]. The most important hepatic lesions involved in these sinusoidal changes are deposition of collagen in the space of Disse, producing a true capillarization of hepatic sinusoids [10], and compression due to enlargement of hepatocytes, particularly when hepatic distensibility is reduced because of diffuse fibrosis [11]. This latter hypothesis, however, is doubtful since there are many experimental studies in disagreement with this concept [12–14].

In the experimental model of CCl_4-induced cirrhosis it has been found that vascular obstruction only appears when hepatic cirrhosis is well established, while portal pressure is already elevated in a pre-cirrhotic stage [15, 16]. This finding has been related to an increase in vascular tone. It is also possible that neurohumoral factors may mediate an active obstruction to portal flow by stimulating the hepatic nerves in these experimental conditions [17]. More recently, it has been suggested that this active component can be due, in part, to the contraction and relaxation of fat-storing cells. Located in the sinusoid, these cells have the ability to contract since they contain actin-like filaments with contractile properties. Consequently, some vasoactive substances, either vasodilators or vasoconstrictors, may modify intrahepatic vascular resistance through relaxiocontraction of these fat-storing cells [18].

The concept that neurohumoral factors may mediate an active obstruction to portal flow in cirrhosis was established in 1961 [19]. At that time it was suggested that the release of adrenaline and noradrenaline to the portal venous blood from the splanchnic sympathetic nerves may contribute to the development of portal hypertension in hepatic cirrhosis. This hypothesis was practically forgotten over the years. Later on, it was demonstrated that noradrenaline plasma levels are very high in decompensated cirrhosis and the hypothesis that neurohumoral factors may be involved in the development of portal hypertension has again arisen. Other vasoconstrictor factors such as angiotensin II and vasopressin have also been suggested as substances that are able to increase intrahepatic vascular resistance [20]. In fact, the administration of alpha-adrenergic agonists (prazosin) and beta-adrenergic antagonists (isoproterenol) reduces intrahepatic vascular resistance, suggesting that adrenergic receptors may be involved in the regulation of intrahepatic vascular resistance [21,22].

Recently, it has been indicated that endothelin may also play an important role in mediating this intrahepatic vascular resistance [23]. Endothelin comprises a family of homologous 21-amino acid peptides (ET-1, ET-2 and ET-3) [24]. Most reported data are related to ET-1 which has powerful vasoconstrictor properties. Specific endothelin receptors are divided into two types: ET(A) receptor and ET(B) receptor [25]. The ET(A) receptor is localized in the vascular smooth muscle and modulates vasoconstrictor effects [26]. The ET(B) receptor is present in a variety of cells including endothelial cells, in which it mediates the release of nitric oxide (NO) [27], a powerful vasodilator [28]. Patients with cirrhosis have high levels of circulating plasma ET-1 [29]. The exact mechanism producing an increase in ET-1 is poorly understood. However, at present, it has been proposed that increased release of ET-1 may be due to the activation of some cytokines (transforming growth factor (TGF-beta) and tumour necrosis factor (TNF)) [29]. In addition, experimental studies have revealed that infusion of ET-1 promotes the contraction of activated fat-storing cells [31] and the closure of the endothelium fenestrae in normal rat liver. These findings are of interest since, as indicated, the capillarization process and occlusion of fenestrae may play a central role in increasing intrahepatic vascular resistance in cirrhosis [32].

When portal hypertension is established, the collateral circulation represents an additional site of increased resistance to portal blood flow [33]. The formation of collaterals probably involves the opening, dilatation and hypertrophy of pre-existing vascular vessels. In addition, active angiogenesis may also be involved in this phenomenon. At present, it is well accepted that the resistance of this collateral bed, although lower than that of the cirrhotic liver, is higher than that of a normal liver [34]. The mechanisms that modulate collateral resistance are not well understood. These vessels are probably more sensitive to serotonin, a substance which increases their vascular resistance. In fact, the administration of selective 5-hydroxytryptamine (5-HT$_2$) receptor blockers to intact portal hypertensive animals produces a decrease in portal pressure without changing systemic haemodynamics and portal flow [35,36]. These findings suggest that portocollateral resistance is partially responsible for the increase in portal pressure. Recent studies performed on isolated perfused portosystemic collateral beds suggest that NO may also be involved in controlling portocollateral vascular resistance [37].

Increased blood flow

Increased blood flow through the portal venous system appears in the advanced stages of portal hypertension, and contributes to the maintenance and aggravation of the portal hypertensive syndrome. The increased portal venous inflow is due to a marked arteriolar vasodilatation in splanchnic organs draining into the portal vein. Therefore, in portal hypertension a vascular territory (portal venous system) simultaneously exhibits increased blood flow and outflow vascular resistance [35,36].

Many mechanisms have been suggested to explain this striking haemodynamic situation, which probably represents a multifactorial phenomenon, and which may involve humoral, neurogenic and local mechanisms. Ten years ago, it was suggested that this haemodynamic abnormality was the consequence of the presence of circulating vasodilators. This concept arose from the fact that cross-circulation studies in portal hypertensive and normal animals demonstrated the development of the splanchnic vasodilation in the recipient, indicating that humoral factors are implicated in splanchnic hyperaemia [38]. At present, several substances such as glucagon, prostacyclin and NO have been implicated.

Glucagon is secreted by pancreatic alpha-cells and the oxyntic gastric mucosa and inactivated by the liver. It is a powerful vasodilator substance and it has been found that plasma glucagon levels are elevated in cirrhotic patients and in experimental models of portal hypertension [38,39]. This hyperglucagonism is mainly due to an increased secretion of pancreatic alpha-cells rather than to a decreased hepatic clearance of glucagon [40,41]. In experimental studies it has been shown that by increasing the circulating glucagon in normal rats to levels similar to those observed in portal hypertensive animals a significant increase may be detected in splanchnic blood flow. Conversely, the normalization of circulating glucagon, in an experimental model of portal hypertension, using somatostatin infusions, partially reverses the increased splanchnic blood flow [39,40]. This response was blocked by preventing the fall in circulating glucagon by a concomitant glucagon infusion [42]. As a consequence of these studies it has been suggested that hyperglucagonism may account for approximately 30–40% of splanchnic vasodilatation in portal hypertension [38]. It is important to take into account that the vasodilatory effects of hyperglucagonism seem to be preferential in the splanchnic circulation with blunted response in systemic circulation. Glucagon may produce vasodilatation by relaxing the vascular smooth muscle and by decreasing the sensitivity to endogenous vasoconstrictors (noradrenaline, angiotensin II, vasopressin) [43,44]. It is considered that these vasoactive effects may be mediated through the activation of adenyl cyclase with a consequent increase in cyclic adenosine monophosphate (cAMP). Other studies, however, have shown divergent results, indicating that in experimental models portal hypertension is not necessarily associated with a high level of circulating glucagon [45].

Prostacyclin is an endogenous vasodilator, produced by vascular endothelial cells, which induces vascular smooth-muscle relaxation by activating adenylate cyclase and increasing the intracellular level of cAMP [46]. Several studies have suggested that prostacyclin may play a role in the hyperdynamic circulation of portal hypertension [47–49]. Thus, it has been shown that cirrhotic patients may have increased plasma levels of prostacyclin [49]. In addition, in portal hypertensive animals it has been found that portal vein levels of prostacyclin are elevated [48]. Furthermore, the inhibition of prostacyclin synthesis by indomethacin reduces the hyperdynamic circulation and portal pressure in cirrhotic patients and portal hypertension [50]. These findings suggest that prostacyclin may play a role in the development of splanchnic vasodilatation in portal hypertension.

Nitric oxide is a secretory product of mammalian cells that is formed from molecular oxygen and the guanidino nitrogen of L-arginine. Among

other numerous biological effects, NO is the natural ligand for soluble guanylate cyclase with a subsequent increase in levels of guanosine 3',5'-cyclic
monophosphate, the final substance responsible for relaxation in the vascular wall [51]. The production of NO is catalysed by the enzyme NO-synthase, of which there are at least three different types in vascular tissue. One is
constitutive and Ca^{2+}/calmodulin-dependent. The other two are inducible by
cytokines   and   bacterial   lipopolysaccharide   and   are Ca^{2+} calmo-
dulin-independent. The constitutive NO-synthase has been cloned in
endothelial cells [52], whereas the inducible isoforms have been identified in
smooth-muscle cells [53]. The activity of these enzymes can be inhibited by
L-arginine analogues such as N(w)-nitro-L-arginine and N(g)-nitro-L-arginine
and N(g)-nitro-L-arginine methyl ester.

Closed interactions exist between the endogenous vasoconstrictors
angiotensin II, noradrenaline and endothelin 1 and endothelial NO release. In
addition to the stimulatory effect of endothelin 1 on NO [27], it appears that
NO is the natural antagonist of angiotensin II, noradrenaline and endothelin
1. On the other hand, NO-synthase inhibition increases the vasopressor
response to these vasoconstrictor agents. These findings are consistent with
the modulatory effect of NO on the vascular action of angiotensin II,
noradrenaline and endothelin 1.

It has recently been suggested that excessive NO production may be
involved in the mechanism of the hyperdynamic circulation associated with
portal hypertension [54–57]. This hypothesis has been suggested by the
results obtained in experimental studies using specific NO inhibitors. In fact,
the acute administration of these specific antagonists provoked splanchnic
and systemic vasoconstriction in portal hypertensive animals and therefore
attenuated the hyperdynamic circulation in these animals. The vasoconstrictor effect of NO inhibition was significantly higher in portal hypertensive
animals than in control animals, suggesting that an excessive amount of NO
may be responsible for the vasodilatation observed in portal hypertension.
Furthermore, NO inhibition is able to correct the characteristic vascular
hyporesponsiveness to vasoconstrictors that is present in portal hypertension
and that is thought to contribute to systemic and splanchnic vasodilatation.
However, it has also been shown that NO inhibition attenuates, although
does not normalize, the hyperkinetic syndrome of portal hyptertension [58,
59]. In addition, a recent study has indicated that chronic NO inhibition,
although able to preclude the development of systemic vasodilatation,
delayed, but did not prevent, the development of splanchnic vasodilatation
[60–62]. These data suggest that factors other than NO are also involved in
the pathogenesis of the hyperdynamic circulation in portal hypertension [62].

Whether the increased NO activity observed in portal hypertension is due
to a hyperstimulation of the constitutive NO-synthase or, as has also been

suggested, to the 'novo' formation of an inducible NO-synthase, still remains controversial [63]. Initially, it was proposed that endotoxaemia, which is frequently observed in cirrhosis, would be able to induce the expression of the inducible NO-synthase [56]. The recent observation that the injection of anti-TNF antibodies attenuates the hyperkinetic circulation in portal hypertension supports this hypothesis [64]. However, the administration of dexamethasone, an inhibitor of the inducible NO-synthase, while preventing the expression of the inducible NO-synthase caused by endotoxin injection, failed to modify the hyperdynamic state of partial portal vein-ligated rats [65]. All this suggests that it is possible that the constitutive NO-synthase which is activated by circulating vasoactive factors such as angiotensin II, noradrenaline and endothelin 1, could also represent an important source for an increased release of NO in portal hypertension.

Other vasodilators have also been involved in the pathogenesis of splanchnic vasodilatation such as bile acids, neuropeptides, adenosine, endotoxin and a variety of vasodilatory gastrointestinal hormones. However, available evidence is scarce for the majority [66,67].

All these data suggest that none of these vasoactive factors (glucagon, prostacyclin and NO) is the only factor responsible for the splanchnic vasodilatation present in portal hypertension, which is likely to be multi-factorial in origin. In addition, experimental studies suggest that when one of these vasoactive mediators, such as prostaglandins [68] or NO [62], is chronically inhibited, other vasoactive pathways may be enhanced preventing the correction of splanchnic vasodilatation. This suggests that there is an interrelationship between these vasoactive systems, which are coupled to cause splanchnic vasodilatation.

Increased plasma volume

It is well established that portal hypertension induces several changes in systemic circulation, the most important being peripheral vasodilatation, expanded plasma volume and hyperkinetic circulation.

The hyperkinetic circulation is characterized by a decrease in arteriolar resistance and by an increase in systemic and regional blood flows. It has been considered that this hyperkinetic circulation is a consequence of an intense vasodilatation that may be induced, as indicated above, by several vasodilator substances. However, this vasodilatation is not the only alteration necessary for the development of this hyperdynamic circulation, since, although pharmacological vasodilators reduce peripheral resistance, they also produce an increase in vascular underfilling. This does not induce any change in systemic blood flow, including cardiac output [69,70]. Nevertheless, increased plasma volume may play an important role in the development of the hyperdynamic circulation. In fact, in the model of partial portal vein-ligated rats it has been demonstrated that sodium intake restriction blunts the development of plasma volume expansion and ameliorates the hyperdynamic circulation [70]. These findings suggest that increased plasma volume plays an important role in the development of high cardiac output and hyperkinetic syndrome associated with portal hypertension. Therefore, it is possible that an increased plasma volume contributes to maintain, and probably to aggravate, portal hypertension. This hypothesis has been confirmed in the model of partial portal vein-ligated rats and in cirrhotic patients. In fact, a low-sodium diet induces the significant reduction of hepatic venous pressure gradient and the administration of diuretics (e.g. spironolactone) also produces a significant reduction of portal pressure [70,71]. These results are also consistent with the hypothesis that increased portal blood flow plays an important role in the maintenance of portal hypertension.

REFERENCES

1 McIndoe AH. Vascular lesions of portal cirrhosis. *Arch Pathol* 1928; 5: 23–42.
2 Ketly RH, Baggenstoss AH, Butt HR. The relation of the regenerated liver nodule to the vascular bed in cirrhosis. *Gastroenterology* 1959; 15: 285–295.
3 Bosch J, García-Pagán JC, Feu F, Rodés J. Portal hypertension. Clinical pathobiology. In: Arias IM, Boyer JL, Fausto N, Jacoby WB, Schachter DA, Shafritz DA (eds) *The Liver, Biology and Pathobiology*. New York: Raven Press, 1994: 1343–1354.
4 Bosch J, Navasa M, García-Pagán JC, De Lacy AM, Rodés J. Portal hypertension. *Med Clin North Am* 1989; 73: 931–953.
5 Bioulac-Sage P, Le Bail B, Balabaud C. Liver and biliary tract histology. In: McIntyre N, Benhamou JP, Bircher J, Rizzetto M, Rodés J (eds), *Oxford Textbook of Clinical Hepatology*. Oxford: Oxford University Press, 1991: 12–20.
6 Gendrault JL, Steffan AM, Bingen A, Kirn A. Kupffer and endothelial cells. In: Bioulac-Sage P, Balabaud C (eds), *Sinusoids in Human Liver: Health and Disease*. Rijswijk: The Kupffer Cell Foundation, 1988: 17–38.
7 Grossman HJ, Grossman VL, Bathal PS. Intrahepatic vascular resistance in cirrhosis. In: Bosch J, Groszmann RJ (eds), *Portal Hypertension. Pathophysiology and Treatment*. Oxford: Blackwell Scientific Publications, 1994: 1–16.
8 Mitzner W. Hepatic outflow resistance, sinusoidal pressure, and the vascular waterfall. *Am J Physiol* 1974; 227: 513–519.
9 Greenway CV, Lautt WW. Distensibility of hepatic venous resistance sites and consequences on portal pressure. *Am J Physiol* 1988; 254: H452–H458.
10 Schaffner F, Popper H. Capillarization of hepatic sinusoids in man. *Gastroenterology* 1963; 44: 239–242.
11 Orrego H, Blendis LM, Crossley IR *et al*. Correlation of intrahepatic pressure with collagen in the Disse space and hepatomegaly in humans and in the rat. *Gastroenterology* 1981; 80: 546–556.
12 Mastai R, Huet PM, Brault A, Belgiorno J. The rat liver microcirculation in alcohol-induced hepatomegaly. *Hepatology* 1989; 10: 941–945.

13 Dagenais M, Giroux L, Belgiorno J, Huet PM. The effect of alcohol-induced hepato-megaly on portal hypertension in cirrhotic rats. *J Hepatol* 1992; **15**: 88–93.

14 Grossman JH, Grossman VL, Bhathal PS. Intrahepatic vascular resistance in cirrhosis. In: Bosch J, Groszman RJ (eds) *Portal Hypertension, Pathophysiology and Treatment.* Oxford: Blackwell Scientific Publications, 1994: 1–16..

15 Reynolds TB, Hidemura R, Michel H, Peters R. Portal hypertension without cirrhosis in alcoholic liver disease. *Ann Intern Med* 1969; **70**: 497–506.

16 van Leuwen DJ, Howe SC, Scheuer PJ, Sherlock S. Portal hypertension in chronic hepatitis: relationship to morphological changes. *Gut* 1990; **31**: 339–343.

17 Krogsgaard K, Gluud C, Henrikson JH, Christifferson P. Correlation between liver morphology and portal pressure in alcoholic liver disease. *Hepatology* 1984; **4**: 699–703.

18 Rockey DC, Housset CN, Friedman SL. Contractility of hepatic lipocytes: implications for the pathogenesis of portal hypertension. *Hepatology* 1992; **16**: 123A.

19 Shaldon C, Peacock JH, Walker RM, Palmer DB, Badrick RE. The portal venous content of adrenaline and noradrenaline in portal hypertension. *Lancet* 1961; **1**: 957–961.

20 Willett IR, Esler M, Jennings G, Dudley FJ. Sympathetic tone modulates portal venous pressure in alcoholic cirrhosis. *Lancet* 1986; **2**: 939–943.

21 Lautt WW, Greenway CV, Legare DJ. Effects of hepatic nerves, norepinephrine, angiotensin, elevated central venous pressure on postsinusoidal resistance sites and intrahepatic pressures. *Microcirculation* 1987; **33**: 50–61.

22 Marteau P, Ballet F, Chazouillères O *et al.* Effects of vasodilators on hepatic micro-circulation in cirrhosis: a study in the isolated perfused rat liver. *Hepatology* 1989; **9**: 820–823.

23 Jiménez W, Rodés J. Impaired responsiveness to endogenous vasoconstrictors and endothelium derived vasoactive factors in cirrhosis. *Gastroenterology* 1994; **107**: 1201–1202.

24 Battistini B, D'Orleans-Juste P, Sirois P. Biology of disease. Endothelins: circulating levels and presence in other biologic fluids. *Lab Invest* 1993; **68**: 600–619.

25 Sakurai T, Yanagisawa M, Masaki T. Molecular characterization of endothelin receptors. *Trends Pharmacol Sci* 1992; **13**: 103–108.

26 Alberts GF, Peifley KA, Johns A, Kleha JF, Winkles JA. Constitutive endothelin-1 overexpression promotes smooth muscle cell proliferation via an external autocrine loop. *J Biol Chem* 1994; **269**, 10112–10118.

27 Hirata Y, Emori T, Eguchi T, Kanno K, Imai T, Ohta K, Marumo F. Endothelin receptor subtype B mediates synthesis of nitric oxide by cultured bovine endothelial cells. *J Clin Invest* 1993; **91**: 1367–1371.

28 Moncada S, Palmer RMJ, Higgs EA. Nitric oxide: physiology, pathophysiology and pharmacology. *Pharmacol Rev* 1991; **43**: 109–142.

29 Asbert M, Ginés A, Ginés P *et al.* Circulating levels of endothelin in cirrhosis. *Gastroenterology* 1993; **104**: 1485–1491.

30 Kamath PS, Miller VM, Tyce GM *et al.* Hepatic endothelin-1 increases vascular resistance in portal hypertension. *J Hepatol* 1994; **21**: S41.

31 Sakamoto M, Ueno T, Kin M *et al.* Ito cell contraction in response to endothelin-1 and substance P. *Hepatology* 1992; **18**: 978–983.

32 Reichen J, Sägesser H. The effect of endothelin on microvascular exchange in rat liver: reversible capillarization by closure of endothelial fenestrae. *J Hepatol* 1994; **21**: S8.

33 Chojkier M, Groszmann RJ. Measurement of portal-systemic shunting in the rat by using labelled microspheres. *Am J Physiol* 1981; **240**: G371–G375.

34 Mosca P, Lee FY, Kaumann AJ et al. Pharmacology of portal-systemic collaterals in portal hypertensive rats: role of endothelium. *Am J Physiol* 1992; **263**: G544–G550.

35 Cummings SA, Groszmann RJ, Kaumann AJ. Hypersensitivity of mesenteric veins to 5-hydroxytryptamine and ketanserin-induced reduction of portal pressure in portal hypertensive rats. *Br J Pharmacol* 1986; **89**: 501–513.

36 Kaumann AJ, Morgan J, Groszmann RJ. ICI 139,369 selectively blocks 5-hydroxytryptamine 2 receptors and lowers portal pressure in portal hypertensive rats. *Gastroenterology* 1988; **95**: 1601–1605.

37 Benoit JN, Granger DN. Splanchnic hemodynamics in chronic portal venous hypertension. *Semin Liv Dis* 1986; **6**: 287–291.

38 Benoit JN, Barrowman JA, Harper SL et al. Role of humoral factors in the intestinal hyperemia associated with chronic portal hypertension. *Am J Physiol* 1984; **247**: 486–493.

39 Benoit JN, Zimmerman B, Premen AJ et al. Role of glucagon in splanchnic hyperemia of chronic portal hypertension. *Am J Physiol* 1986; **251**: G674–G678.

40 Kravetz D, Bosch J, Arderiu MT et al. Effects of somatostatin on splanchnic hemodynamics and plasma glucagon in portal hypertensive rats. *Am J Physiol* 1988; **254**: G322–G325.

41 Gomis R, Fernández Alvarez J et al. Impaired function of pancreatic islets from rats with portal hypertension resulting from cirrhosis and partial portal vein ligation. *Hepatology* 1994; **19**: 1257–1261.

42 Pizcueta MP, García-Pagán JC, Fernández M et al. Glucagon hinders the effects of somatostatin in portal hypertension. A study in rats with partial portal vein ligation. *Gastroenterology* 1991; **101**: 1710–1715.

43 Pizcueta MP, Casamitjana R, Bosch J et al. Decreased systemic vascular sensitivity to norepinephrine in portal hypertensive rats. Role of hyperglucagonism. *Am J Physiol* 1990; **258**: G191–G194.

44 Richardson PDI, Withrington PG. The inhibition of the vasoconstrictor actions of noradrenaline, angiotensin and vasopressin on the hepatic arterial vascular bed of the dog. *Br J Pharmacol* 1976; **57**: 93–101.

45 Sikuler E, Groszmann RJ. Hemodynamic studies in long and short term portal hypertensive rats: the relation to systemic glucagon levels. *Hepatology* 1986; **6**: 414–418.

46 Smith WL. Prostaglandin biosynthesis and its compartmentation in vascular smooth muscle and endothelial cells. *Ann Rev Physiol* 1986; **48**: 251–262.

47 Sitzmann JV, Bulkley GB, Campbell K et al. Role of prostacyclin in the splanchnic hyperemia contributing to portal hypertension. *Ann Surg* 1989; **209**: 322–327.

48 Hamilton G, Phing RCF, Hutton RA et al. The relationship between prostacyclin activity and pressure in the portal vein. *Hepatology* 1982; **2**: 236–242.

49 Guarner C, Soriano G, Such J et al. Systemic prostacyclin in cirrhotic patients: relationship with portal hypertension and changes after intestinal decontamination. *Gastroenterology* 1992; **102**: 303–309.

50 Bruix J, Bosch J, Kravetz D et al. Effects of prostaglandin inhibition on systemic and hepatic hemodynamics in patients with cirrhosis of the liver. *Gastroenterology* 1985; **88**: 430–435.

51 Nathan C. Nitric oxide as a secretory product of mammalian cells. *FASEB J* 1992; **6**: 3051–3064.

52 Lamas S, Marsden PA, Li GK, Tempst P, Michel T. Endothelial nitric oxide synthase:

molecular cloning and characterization of a distinct constitutive enzyme isoform. *Proc Natl Acad Sci USA* 1992; **89**: 6348–6352.

53 Nunokawa Y, Ishida N, Tanaka S. Cloning of inducible nitric oxide synthase in rat vascular smooth muscle cells. *Biochem Biophys Res Commun* 1993; **1991**: 89–94.

54 Pizcueta MP, Piqué JM, Fernández M *et al*. Modulation of the hyperdynamic circulation of cirrhotic rats by nitric oxide inhibition. *Gastroenterology* 1992; **103**: 1909–1915.

55 Pizcueta MP, Piqué JM, Bosch J *et al*. Effects of inhibiting nitric oxide biosynthesis on the systemic and splanchnic circulation of rats with portal hypertension. *Br J Pharmacol* 1992; **105**: 184–190.

56 Vallance P, Moncada S. Hyperdynamic circulation in cirrhosis: a role for nitric oxide. *Lancet* 1991; **337**: 776.

57 Guarner C, Soriano G, Tomas A *et al*. Increased serum nitrite and nitrate levels in patients with cirrhosis: relationship to endotoxemia. *Hepatology* 1993; **18**: 1139–1143.

58 Sieber CC, Groszmann RJ. Nitric oxide mediates hyporeactivity to vasopressors in mesenteric vessels of portal hypertensive rats. *Gastroenterology* 1992; **103**: 235–239.

59 Lee FY, Albillos A, Colombato L *et al*. The role of nitric oxide in the vascular hyporesponsiveness to methoxamine in portal hypertensive rats. *Hepatology* 1992; **16**: 1043–1048.

60 Lee FX, Colombato LA, Albillos A *et al*. N-Nitro-L-arginine administration corrects peripheral vasodilation and systemic capillary hypotension and ameliorates plasma volume expansion and sodium retention in portal hypertensive rats. *Hepatology* 1993; **17**: 84–90.

61 Lee FY, Colombato LA, Albillos A *et al*. Administration of N-Nitro-L-arginine ameliorates portal system shunting in portal hypertensive rats. *Gastroenterology* 1993; **105**: 1464–1470.

62 García-Pagán JC, Fernández M, Bernadich C *et al*. Effects of continued nitric oxide inhibition on the development of the portal hypertensive syndrome following portal vein stenosis in the rat. *Am J Physiol* 1994; **30**: 984–990.

63 Busse R, Mülsch A, Fleming I, Hecker M. Mechanisms of nitric oxide release from the vascular endothelium. *Circulation* 1993; **87**: V18–V25.

64 López-Talavera JC, Merril W, Groszmann RJ. Treatment with anti-tumor necrosis factor-α polyclonal antibodies prevents the development of the hyperdynamic circulation and reduces portal pressure in portal hypertensive rats. *Hepatology* 1993; **18**: 140A.

65 García-Pagán JC, Fernández M, Casadevall M *et al*. Prevention of the expression of Ca2-independent inducible NO synthase by chronic dexamethasone administration does not modify the hyperdynamic circulation in portal hypertensive rats. *Hepatology* (*in press*).

66 Genecin P, Polio J, Colombato LA *et al*. Bile acids do not mediate the hyperdynamic circulation in portal hypertensive rats. *Am J Physiol* 1990; **259**: G21–G25.

67 Thomas SH, Joh T, Benoit JN. Role of bile acids in splanchnic hemodynamic response to chronic portal hypertension. *Dig Dis Sci* 1991; **36**: 1243–1248.

68 Fernández M, García-Pagán JC, Casadevall M *et al*. Hemodynamic effects of acute and chronic cyclooxygenase inhibition in portal hypertensive rats. Influence of nitric oxide biosynthesis. *Gastroenterology* (*in press*).

69 Pagani M, Vatner ST, Braunwaldt F. hemodynamic effects of intravenous sodium nitroprusiate in the conscious dog. *Circulation* 1978; **57**: 144–157.

70 Genecin P, Polio J, Groszmann RJ. Na restriction blunts expansion of plasma volume and ameliorates hyperdynamic circulation in portal hypertension. *Am J Physiol* 1990; **259**: G498–G503.

71 García-Pagán JC, Salmerón JM, Feu F *et al.* Effects of low sodium diet and spironolactone on portal pressure in patients with compensated cirrhosis. *Hepatology* 1994; **19**: 1095–1099.

Diagnostic Issues: Portal Hypertensive Gastropathy and Gastric Varices

Shiv K. Sarin

I Portal hypertensive gastropathy

Definition

Since the initial description [1,2], portal hypertensive gastropathy (PHG) has come to be defined as unequivocal endoscopic evidence of mosaic-like pattern (MLP) and red markings (RM) in the stomach of a patient with portal hypertension [3]. Histopathologically, mucosal and submucosal vascular dilatation is seen in these patients [4].

Several conditions could transiently alter the endoscopic findings of gastric mucosa [5]; these include: infection with *Helicobacter pylori*, alcoholic gastritis, drug-associated gastritis, post-sclerotherapy changes or a recent bleed from the varices. We therefore recommend that two endoscopies should be performed at least 1 week apart, before accepting a diagnosis of PHG [6]. This approach would also help in decreasing the observer bias. The need for histological confirmation should remain optional except in the course of clinical studies.

DESCRIPTION OF PORTAL HYPERTENSIVE GASTROPATHY LESIONS AND CLASSIFICATION

There was agreement on the description of the two elementary lesions of PHG, namely, MLP (Plates 1 and 2, opposite p. 34) and RM (Plates 3–5, opposite p. 34) at the consensus meeting held at Milan [3]. Since cherry-red spots were found to have overlapping features with red spots, the two terms were merged together and renamed as red markings (RM). Black–brown spots were considered as evidence of an old intramucosal bleed and not different from the RM. However, even in this revised NIEC classification there are difficulties. According to this classification, PHG is *mild* when only MLP is present, and *severe* when RM are present. The classification does not refer to: (i) the grade of MLP – mild (pink), moderate (flat red spots), and severe (diffuse red areola); (ii) the grade of PHG if both MLP and RM are present; or (iii) how to classify severe MLP in the absence of RM. Further, reproducibility of the NIEC classification is poor and MLP lesions are not specific for portal hypertension [3,7–10]. On the other hand, observer variability is low and predictability of bleeding high with RM. Classifications based only on RM have been proposed: *mild PHG* represents isolated RM, and *severe PHG* represents confluent RM. Such a classification was found to be both reproducible [6] and useful [10].

Before we proceed to improve the existing classifications, we should be able to answer a vital question: what is the clinical significance of the two elementary lesions, namely MLP and RM, and how often does overt and occult bleeding occur due to them? The data as provided by the panellists are shown in Table 1. There is a wide variation in the frequency of gastro-intestinal (GI) bleeding from these lesions.

Another important endoscopic lesion seen in portal hypertension patients is gastric antral vascular ectasia (GAVE) (Plate 6, opposite p. 35). This was recognized more than a decade ago as an entity with distinct clinical, endo-scopic and histopathological features [11]. It has been reported in association with scleroderma, atrophic gastritis and cirrhosis of the liver [12]. While it is considered a distinct entity from PHG [13], it is often seen in cirrhotic patients. Calés *et al.* have recently found GAVE in 14 of their 34 patients (37%); the same frequency as of severe PHG. In fact, their patients with GAVE had a significantly lower haemoglobin and increased blood loss [13]. We have observed GAVE in 1.1% of patients with cirrhosis and in 0.5% of those with non-cirrhotic portal hypertension. Because of its common asso-ciation with all types of portal hypertension and frequent associated bleed-ing, we propose that GAVE should be considered as part of the PHG syndrome. Based on these facts we have developed a simple objective classification of PHG (Table 2).

This scoring system would allow objective assessment of each mucosal lesion of PHG. This may be prospectively evaluated.

ASSESSMENT OF BLOOD LOSS

Acute or chronic blood loss is the most common presentation of PHG [10, 13–15]. However, data on the frequency and on the amount of blood loss have been variable (Table 1). A recent study has shown that anaemia and blood loss are not a frequent occurrence in severe PHG, with only ca. 9 ml blood being lost daily from the mucosa in patients with severe PHG [13]. In another recent study, there was no difference in the haemoglobin (Hb) level in patients with or without PHG [14]. On the other hand, some workers have shown that as many as 50–60% of patients with severe PHG bleed

Table 1 Clinical significance (% bleeding) of endoscopic lesions of PHG.*

Reference	No. of patients	MLP		RM		Both		Follow-up (months)
		Occult (%)	Overt (%)	Occult (%)	Overt (%)	Occult (%)	Overt (%)	
Calés et al. [7]		0?	0?	0?	<5?	0?	<5?	
D'Amico et al. [15]	130	30	35	60	90	35	43	46
Sarin et al. [8]								
Cirrhosis	362	—	—	—	1.1	—	1.1	48
Non-cirrhosis	209	—	—	—	0.5	—	0.5	48

* Unpublished data provided in response to questionnaire.
MLP, mosaic-like pattern; RM, red markings.

Table 2 Portal hypertensive gastropathy (PHG) score.

Lesion	Score
Mosaic-like pattern	
Mild	1
Severe	2
Red markings	
Isolated	1
Confluent	2
GAVE	
Absent	0
Present	2
Mild PHG	$\leqslant 3$
Severe PHG	$\geqslant 4$

GAVE, gastric antral vascular ectasia.

significantly [10,15]. Why is there so much discrepancy? Perhaps our methods are insensitive, or have not been used carefully enough to assess blood loss as a result of PHG.

1 It is difficult to assess *correctly* the source of *active* bleeding in a patient with PHG who also has oesophageal/gastric varices. It is not known whether the acute PHG bleed is a slow ooze or an acute massive bleed. A repeat endoscopy should always be performed a few hours or a day later to detect any oozing from PHG lesions [2,6].

2 Reduction of Hb by more than 2 g/dl, in the absence of a variceal bleed, has been considered significant in the diagnosis of chronic mucosal bleeding from PHG. However, it is not easy to assess whether the bleeding is from PHG, intestinal vasculopathy or colopathy. The current methods to assess blood loss from PHG, namely Hb level, serum iron, and ^{51}Cr-labelled red blood cells, can hardly suggest the site of mucosal bleeding.

3 What is the best way to diagnose that anaemia in a patient with cirrhosis that is the result of either chronic blood loss, liver disease *per se*, poor absorption, drug interactions, associated renal disease or bone marrow suppression, etc.?

Until these issues are resolved, different clinical presentations of PHG should continue to be reported.

CLINICAL COURSE AND NATURAL HISTORY OF PORTAL HYPERTENSIVE GASTROPATHY

Two prospective studies [10,15] have shown that PHG is present in more than 50% of cirrhotics. During a mean follow-up of 60 months, significantly more patients with severe (62%) and mild (31%) PHG had overt bleeding compared with patients with portal hypertension but without PHG [15]. However, controversy surrounds these observations, as answers to the following questions are unclear.

1   Is PHG a transient or a persistent lesion? A recent report indicated that in most patients the changes in severity of PHG are reversible [16]. Our experience is similar, especially in patients in whom PHG develops after sclerotherapy.

2   How does one assess progression of PHG?
   (a) Does the MLP change to RM and vice versa?
   (b) Can mild lesions become severe and vice versa?
   (c) Do isolated RM become confluent and vice versa?

Moreover, observer variability is inherent to PHG assessment.

FACTORS INFLUENCING DEVELOPMENT OF PORTAL HYPERTENSIVE GASTROPATHY

Several factors could influence the development of PHG, the most important being the severity of liver disease [10] and endoscopic sclerotherapy [6]. Endoscopic variceal ligation (EVL) has little influence on the development of PHG as compared with sclerotherapy [17] and the changes revert to normal more rapidly than after sclerotherapy [16]. The aetiology of portal hypertension, cirrhotic or non-cirrhotic, also has a bearing. Non-cirrhotic portal hypertension constitutes about 40–50% of all patients with portal hypertension in developing countries such as India. It includes patients with non-cirrhotic portal fibrosis and extrahepatic portal vein obstruction [18]. We have not encountered PHG in non-cirrhotic patients, despite portal pressure comparable with those in cirrhotics [5] unless the patients had undergone sclerotherapy. The exact mechanism of protection of the gastric mucosa in these patients is not clear, but is probably due to the near normal liver function in such cases.

Certain factors could influence induction of bleeding from PHG. The PHG mucosa in rats was found to be more vulnerable to bleeding when exposed to aspirin, alocohol and bile acids [19,20]. There are no human trials to confirm these reports.

PATHOGENESIS

Portal hypertension is a *sine qua non* for the development of PHG. However, there is controversy regarding any direct correlation between the gastric capillary ectasia and the degree of portal hypertension [6,21]. D'Amico *et al.* on the other hand found a correlation between variceal size and severity of PHG [15]. Iwao *et al.* [22] and Ohta *et al.* [14] reported a significant correlation

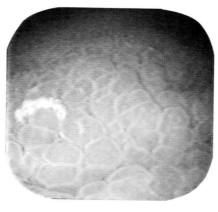

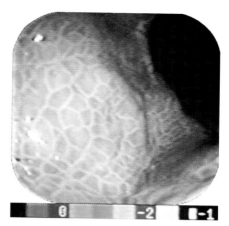

Plate 1 Mosaic-like pattern (MLP) – mild the areola is diffusely pink.

Plate 2 MLP – severe: the areola is diffusely red.

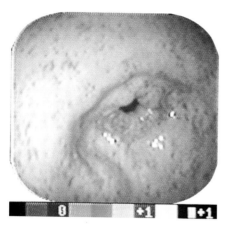

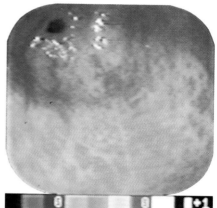

Plate 3 Red marks (RM) – discrete red points.

Plate 4 RM – confluent red points.

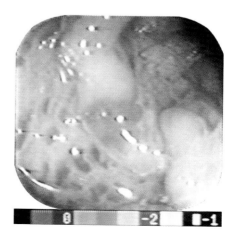

Plate 5 RM – cherry-red spots.

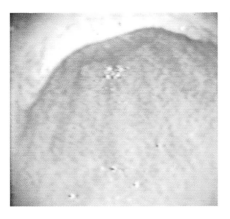

Plate 6 Gastric antral vascular ectasia (GAVE).

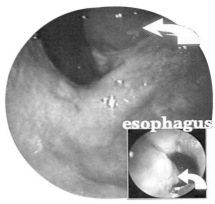

Plate 7 NIEC classification of gastric varices: type 1 – cardial varices in continuity with oesophageal varices.

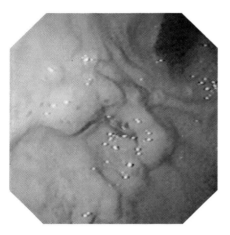

Plate 8 NIEC classification of gastric varices Type 2 – true gastric varices.

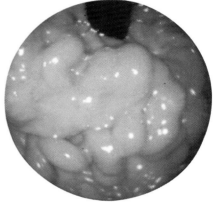

Plate 9 NIEC classification of gastric varices G+: bunch of grapes.

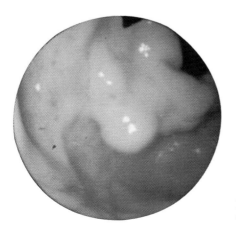

Plate 10 NIEC classification of gastric varices G−: no bunch of grapes.

between the hepatic portal venous pressure gradient and the presence and severity of PHG. In the latter study there was, however, no difference in the portal pressure, oesophageal variceal pressure, portal vein flow and congestion index of the portal vein between patients with and without PHG. Thus, the significance of only one haemodynamic parameter, hepatic vein pressure gradient (HVPG), requires confirmation. Controversy also shrouds the results of gastric mucosal blood flow measurements in patients with PHG. Sarfeh and co-workers [19] and Iwao *et al.* [22] believe that gastric mucosal perfusion is decreased in PHG. This leads to reduced postaglandin production and to a vulnerable gastric mucosa. Iwao *et al.* [23], using laser-Doppler flowmetry and reflectance spectroscopy, have further suggested that there is a 'passive' congestion (stasis) rather than active (overflow) hyperdynamic circulation in PHG mucosa. This is characterized by increased blood volume and decreased perfusion. On the other hand, many investigators have shown that gastric mucosal blood flow is increased in experimental animals [24,25] as well as in cirrhotic patients [26,27] with PHG.

Inflammation of the gastric mucosa does not contribute to the development of PHG [15,28]. The association of *H. pylori* is also lower in severe PHG patients than in the healthy controls [15]. Although low serum pepsinogen levels have been reported in patients with PHG [21], no definite association between atrophic gastritis and PHG has been shown.

Similarly, gastric acid has only a minor role. In fact, its production has been shown to be low in cirrhotic [29] as well as in non-cirrhotic portal hypertension [30]. The gastric intramucosal pH is comparable between cirrhotics and controls [31]. Moreover, there is no response to H_2-receptor antagonists in patients with PHG [1]. The role of antral motility and gastric emptying in patients with PHG is currently being evaluated.

CORRELATION WITH INTESTINAL VASCULOPATHY

Portal hypertension diffusely affects the gastrointestinal tract. It is quite likely that, besides the stomach, the mucosa of the intestines and colon is also affected. There are limited data on the intestinal vasculopathy, though we have recently observed a close correlation between the occurrence of colopathy and PHG [32] (Table 3). While colopathy was a common phenomenon, bleeding from these lesions was seen in only 4% of patients.

CORRELATION WITH GASTRIC VARICES

There are limited data on this aspect. Calés *et al.*, in an anecdotal experience, observed no influence of gastric varices (GV) on the development of PHG. In our prospective study of 107 patients, 36 had coexisting GV and the rest had

Table 3 Influence of gastric varices and colopathy on portal hypertensive gastropathy (PHG).

Parameter	No. of patients	PHG-positive (%)
Gastric varices		
Present	36	42
Absent	71	11
Colopathy		
Present	26	35
Absent	24	8

only oesophageal varices before sclerotherapy. PHG developed in 42% of the former and 11% of the latter patients ($P < 0.01$) [6] (Table 3). This suggests that the chances of development of PHG are increased nearly fourfold if a patient presents with gastro-oesophageal varices (GOV) rather than with oesophageal varices alone. The higher association of PHG with GV could be explained by redistribution and an increase in gastric blood flow after obliteration of oesophageal varices. However, Eleftheriadis *et al.* [33], using endoscopic laser-Doppler technique, found an increase in the gastric microcirculation after sclerotherapy only in the pyloric area, and not in the fundic area, where gastropathy is more common.

THERAPY

The efficacy of treatment for PHG should be assessed by at least two parameters, namely control of bleeding and regression of the endoscopic lesions.

Emergency control of portal hypertensive gastropathy bleeding

In the only controlled study in patients presenting with acute bleeding, propranolol successfully controlled bleeding in six of 12 patients (50%), while placebo controlled bleeding in two of 12 (17%) patients ($P < 0.05$) [10]. Anecdotal data are available on the use of somatostatin and glypressin in acute PHG bleeding. While success rates of up to 85% have been claimed with both (G. Amico and S.A. Jenkins, unpublished data), somatostatin may be marginally better due to its ability to suppress glucagon secretion.

Elective treatment

In the initial uncontrolled studies it was shown that by decreasing portal pressure and portal blood flow, propranolol could decrease the frequency of bleeding from PHG [34]. In another trial, propranolol was found to prevent rebleeding during long-term follow-up [10]. A significantly higher percentage of patients remained bleed-free at 12 months compared with controls (65 vs. 38%; $P < 0.05$). Contrary to expectations, the same authors did not find propranolol superior to placebo in improving the gastric mucosal lesions [10].

Fifty per cent of cirrhotic patients with PHG experienced rebleeding during a 2-year period of follow-up [10]. Whether a combination of propranolol and nitrates could be better than propranolol alone remains to be seen; we are awaiting the results of the European multicentric clinical trial.

Histopathologically, PHG lesions resemble gastrointestinal angiodysplasia. In the latter condition, a combination of oestrogen and progesterone has been found to be useful in controlling bleeding [35]. In an experimental study, the hormonal combination was shown to decrease the gastric mucosal hyperaemia, mucosal vessel density and portal pressure by increasing the portocollateral resistance in portal hypertensive rats [36]. It was proposed that the oestrogen–progesterone combination decreases the gastric mucosal blood flow by counteracting the hyporesponsiveness of the chronically hypertensive gastric vasculature. A reduction of the angiogenesis was an additional mechanism proposed.

Transjugular intrahepatic portosystemic shunt (TIPS)

There is limited experience with TIPS in patients with bleeding PHG.

Surgery

The role of decompressive surgery has been adequately analysed (Table 4). It is clear that a reduction in portal pressure decreases the chances of development and progression of PHG. On the other hand, devascularization may increase the chances of bleeding from PHG (G. Battaglia, personal communication).

Liver transplantation

Orthotopic liver transplant has been found to be quite effective for the treatment of PHG (Table 4). However, transplant at present should be reserved only for refractory and severe PHG bleeds.

Prophylactic treatment of portal hypertensive gastropathy lesions

It has been argued that a significant proportion of patients with portal hypertension develop PHG and more than 50% of them bleed; indeed, 15% bleed quite severely. More alarming is the fact that, of those who bleed once,

Table 4 Influence of surgery on portal hypertensive gastropathy PHG.*

Reference	No. of patients	Mild		Moderate		Severe	
		Presurgery (%)	Postsurgery (%)	Presurgery(%)	Postsurgery (%)	Presurgery (%)	Postsurgery (%)
Gerunda et al.							
Shunt	?	63	29	57	32	14	5
OLT	56	8	0	58	0	32	0
Battaglia et al.							
Shunt	520	?	0	?	0	?	0

* Unpublished data provided by panellists.
OLT, orthotopic liver transplantation.

the chances of rebleeding are 62% at 1 year [10], a figure quite close to the frequency of variceal rebleeding. With such a high proportion of PHG bleeding, would it be advisable to treat all PHG patients with prophylactic beta-blockers? There may, however, be a need for caution, since at present: (i) the data for the frequency of bleeding from PHG are very variable; (ii) propranolol is not tolerated by every patient; and (iii) propranolol is successful in preventing PHG-related bleed in only about 50% of cases. It would thus be premature to give propranol to every patient with PHG. There is, however, a case for giving propranolol to such patients who are alcoholic and are non-abstinent or to those who require regular aspirin or other non-steroidal anti-inflammatory drugs (NSAIDs).

In conclusion, although our understanding of portal hypertensive gastropathy has increased over the past 5 years, there remain many aspects of this entity which are shrouded in controversy. However, this is exactly the case for variceal bleeding and many other diseases in medicine. Attempts to resolve such controversies would promote more innovative and careful work in the future.

II Gastric varices

By logic, any varix present in the stomach should be termed a gastric varix. There is great variability in the reported prevalence of GV [37–40], such discrepancies being due to: (i) difficulty in the diagnosis; (ii) differences in the classification; and (iii) the stage of portal hypertension when a patient is examined for gastric or oesophageal varices. In our experience of 568 consecutive patients with portal hypertensionn [41], primary GV (varices detected at the initial presentation) were seen in 114 (20%) patients. They were significantly more common in bleeders than in non-bleeders (27 vs. 4%; $P < 0.001$). A prevalence of 19.7% of GV has been reported from the NIEC group (unpublished data, 1995).

DIAGNOSIS OF GASTRIC VARICES

Endoscopy remains the mainstay of diagnosis of GV. While observer variability in the diagnosis of oesophageal varices is small, this is not true for GV. Full inflation of the stomach and proper inspection of the fundus and duodenum is mandatory. Despite this, in a small proportion of patients the diagnosis remains 'probable' [41]. To confirm these 'probable' cases, we advise a repeat endoscopy and concurrence of two experienced endoscopists. There should then be little justification to label 'probable' GV, as indicated in the NIEC classification.

While splenoportography can delineate the gastric wall collaterals very well, it cannot suggest the proximity of GV to gastric mucosa, or in other words, the likelihood of bleeding.

Endosonography [43] is increasingly used for enhancing the detection of GV; however, its use is limited by technical difficulties.

CLASSIFICATION

Several classifications have been proposed for GV [3,39,41,42,44] (Table 5). While the first two classifications are based on shape, the next two are based on location. The NIEC and the Hashizume's classifications are based on location, form and mucosal lesions. Although more comprehensive, both are complicated, overlapping and have certain limitations.

1   The direction of the subcardial veins has not been specified; it could be on the lesser curve or on the greater curve towards the fundus. A differentiation in the veins going in the two directions has been shown to be important.

Table 5 Classification of gastric varices.

I Hosking et al. (1988) [39]

Type 1: varices which appear as an inferior extension of oesophageal varices across squamocolumnar junction

Type 2: gastric varices (nearly always accompanied by oesophageal varices) located in the fundus, which appear to converge towards the cardia

Type 3: gastric varices located in the fundus or body in the absence of oesophageal varices and which appear unconnected to the cardia

II Sarin et al. [41]

GASTRO-OESOPHAGEAL VARICES (GOV)

These varices extend beyond the gastro-oesophageal junction and are always associated with oesophageal varices. Further subdivided into:

Type 1 (GOV1): these appear as continuation of oesophageal varices and extend for 2–5 cm below the grastro-oesophageal junction along the lesser curve of the stomach. They are more or less straight

Type 2 (GOV2): these varices extend beyond the grastro-oesophageal junction into the fundus of the stomach. These are long and tortuous

ISOLATED GASTRIC VARICES (IGV)

Gastric varices in the absence of oesophageal varices or 'isolated GV'

Type 1 (IGV1): these varices are located in the fundus of the stomach and fall short of the cardia by a few centimetres

Type 2 (IGV2): these include 'ectopic varices' present in the stomach or duodenum

The GV could be *primary* (present at the initial presentation) or *secondary* (appear after sclerotherapy for oesophageal varices).

Continued

Table 5 Continued.

III Hashizume et al. (1990) [44]

FACTORS	SUBTYPE
Colour (C)	Cw: white or blueish
	Cr: red
Red-colour spots (Rc)	Rc(−): none
	RC(+): present
Form (F)	F1: tortuous, winding
	F2: nodular, small to moderate
	F3: tumourous, huge
Location (L)	La: locus anterior
	L1: locus lesser curvature
	Lp: locus posterior
	Lg: locus greater curvature
	Lf: locus fundic

IV NIEC [3]

TYPE

Type 0 (possible gastric varices): when there are doubts regarding endoscopic identification between folds and small gastric varices

Type 1 (cardial–oesophageal varices or cardial varices in continuity with oesophageal varices) (Plate 7, opposite p. 35)

Type 2 (true gastric varices, fundic and/or cardial) (Plate 8, opposite p. 35): they are localized in the fundus and/or the cardial area and can extend to the body

FORM

Bunch of grapes (G+) (Plate 9, opposite p. 35): so-called pseudotumoural or huge varices

No bunch of grapes (G-) (Plate 10, opposite p. 35): nodular-shaped varices; they can be seen on the wall of the stomach, when the stomach is inflated

---

2 The reported frequency of mucosal lesions over GV is quite variable; only in one of 25 (4%) patients in a recent NIEC analysis of 167 patients (G. Battaglia, unpublished data). In contrast, mucosal lesions were reported in 36% of patients by Hashizume et al. [44]. However, these latter workers showed that patients with RM had bled significantly more than those without them (52 vs. 13.6%). They believe that these lesions only help to indicate a recent bleed rather than in predicting future GV bleeds.

3 Should F2 be differentiated from F3 varices when the two bleed similarly, albeit F3 slightly less than F2?

4 Further, the NIEC and Hashizume's classifications do not differentiate between primary (at first presentation) and secondary (developing after sclerotherapy for oesophageal varices) GV.

What should our aim be in classifying GV? Should the stress be on the appearance of the veins or on the identification of GV at high risk of bleeding?

It is important first to know the natural history of different types of GV.

The data presented below are based on our classification (Fig. 1) used in the prospective study of 568 patients with reference to other published reports on GV.

NATURAL HISTORY OF GASTRIC VARICES

Patients with GV generally present either with recurrent episodes of GV bleeding or with hepatic encephalopathy.

Profile of gastric variceal bleeding

The source of bleeding may remain obscure in up to 50% of patients with GV at the time of their first bleed [45]. Bleeding should be considered to have arisen from GV if: (i) an active bleed or ooze is seen from the GV; (ii) a clot or blackish ulcer is seen on the GV; or (iii) in the presence of distinct large GV and absence of oesophageal varices, no other cause of upper gastrointestinal (UGI) bleeding is detectable [46].

The exact mechanism of rupture of GV is not known. The GV are covered with relatively thick gastric mucosa, and their pressure is relatively lower than that in oesophageal varices [40]. In fact, portal pressure in patients with

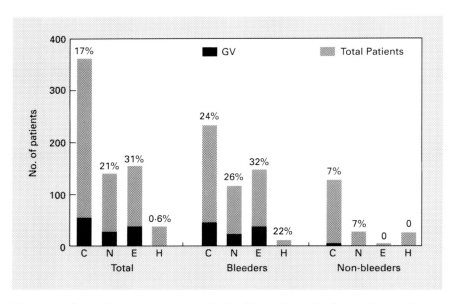

Fig. 1 Prevalence of gastric varices (GV) in bleeding and non-bleeding patients with different pathogeneses of portal hypertension. C, cirrhosis; N, non-cirrhotic portal fibrosis; E, extrahepatic portal vein occlusion; H, hepatic vein outflow obstruction. (Reproduced from Sarin *et al.*, *Hepatology* 1992; **16**: 1343.)

GV bleeding was lower than in non-bleeders (25.2 ± 6.2 vs. 32.4 ± 7.1 cmH_2O, $P < 0.01$).

There are conflicting reports on how often and how severely GV bleed. Terés et al. [47] have reported an incidence of 14–16% bleeding from GV. Paquet [48] observed GV in 60–70% of patients with portal hypertension, and bleeding from fundal varices in 3% of patients. Weissberg et al. [49] found bleeding from varices milder and less common. While 52% of patients bleeding from oesophageal varices died in their series, only 20% with bleeding from GV died ($P < 0.03$). Bretagne et al. [50], on the other hand, found bleeding from GOV more severe and fatal than from oesophageal varices. Calés et al. feel that bleeding occurs from GV in one of every six patients (unpublished data, 1995). In a prospective study of 393 consecutive variceal bleeders [41], we found that the mean number of bleeding episodes before presentation were comparable in patients with GV and oesophageal varices (2.14 ± 1.03 vs. 2.3 ± 1.8). The bleeding risk factor per year (total number of bleeding episodes/time interval between the first and last bleed) for oesophageal varices was higher than for GV (4.3 ± 0.4 vs. 2.0 ± 0.6, $P < 0.01$). However, the mean blood transfusion requirements in GV bleeds were significantly more than for oesophageal variceal bleeds (4.8 ± vs. 2.9 ± 0.3 transfusion units, $P < 0.01$). These data suggest that GV bleed less frequently but more severely than oesophageal varices.

It is also important to know the bleeding profile of different types of GV. Except for our own study, there is limited information in the literature. Hence, I would use our classification (Fig. 2). The prevalence of different types of GV, based upon our classification, is illustrated in Fig. 2. Figure 3 depicts the frequency of bleeding in various types of GV. It is clear that IGV1 and GOV type 2 (GOV2) types of varices have a high incidence of bleeding and hence require careful management. A higher incidence of bleeding from fundic varices has also been reported by other workers [51–53].

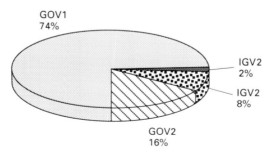

Fig. 2 Relative frequency (%) of different types of primary GV (Sarin classification [41]). (Reproduced from Sarin and Lahoti, *Baillière's Clin Gastroenterol* 1992; **6**: 527.)

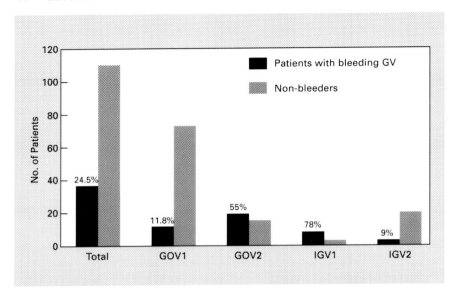

Fig. 3 Frequency of bleeding from different types of GV (Sarin classification [41]). The percentages shown indicate the proportion of total patients with GV who bled. (Reproduced from Sarin and Lahoti, *Baillière's Clin Gastroenterol* 1992; **6**: 527.)

Influence of oesophageal variceal sclerotherapy

This has been studied under the following three groups.

1 Influence of oesophageal variceal sclerotherapy on the fate of coexisting gastric varices

Only GOV are likely to be influenced in this manner.

(a) Gastro-oesophageal varices type I (GOV1): in our prospective study, 78 patients with GOV1, presenting with oesophageal variceal bleeding underwent sclerotherapy. Gastric varices disappeared concurrently or within 6 months (mean ± SEM 4.6 ± 0.42 months) of obliteration of the oesophageal varices in 46 (59%) patients. However, in 32 (41%) patients, GOV1 persisted. Similar observations have been reported by other workers [54]. In fact, Takase *et al.* [55] and Jorge *et al.* [56] have recommended injecting a large volume of sclerosant into the oesophageal varices to achieve obliteration of these veins.

(b) Disappearing vs. persisting GOV1: bleeding was more common in patients in whom GOV1 persisted for more than 6 months after oesophageal sclerotherapy than in those in whom the GV were to disappear (28 vs. 2%, $P < 0.01$) [41]. Similar observations of high bleeding from persisting GV are reported by other workers [51].

(c) GOV2: oesophageal variceal sclerotherapy only marginally influences the treatment of GOV2. Of our 18 patients who received oesophageal variceal sclerotherapy, GOV2 disappeared in only three (17%) patients within 6 months.

Thus, in our experience, three of five patients with GOV1 do not require any treatment except sclerotherapy for oesophageal varices. Close endoscopic observation is, however, advisable to see if the GOV1 persist, since such patients would require gastric variceal sclerotherapy. Most of the patients with GOV2 require direct and specific therapy. In general, we recommend that in a patient with GOV, be it GOV1 or GOV2, initially, only oesophageal varices should be injected.

2 Development of secondary gastric varices

Gastric varices do develop after obliteration of oesophageal varices. The reported frequencies vary between 8.8% [41], 10% [39] and 57% [53]. The discrepancies in the reported series could be due to differences in the patient populations or the time when the patients were observed. In the majority of our patients, secondary GV were GOV2 or IGV2 in type. While the secondary GOV1 and IGV2 types of varices rarely bleed, the frequency of bleeding in patients with secondary GOV2 was similar to that of primary GOV2. These patients therefore require specific therapy.

3 Induction of bleeding from gastric varices

Bleeding from GV due to oesophageal variceal sclerotherapy is quite rare. An incidence of 1–10% reported in the literature seems to be too high [57].

HEPATIC ENCEPHALOPATHY

Cirrhotics with GV develop encephalopathy more often than patients with only oesophageal varices (25 vs. 3%) [40]. This is due to the entry of nitrogenous substances from the gut directly into the systemic circulation through the shunts which form the GV. This, however, is not true for patients with non-cirrhotic portal hypertension, who despite having a higher reported incidence of GV [41] do not have an increased incidence of hepatic ence-phalopathy [58].

PATHOGENESIS AND ORIGIN OF GASTRIC VARICES

Lesser curve GV (GOV1) form because one of the branches of the left gastric vein perpendicularly perforates the gastric wall and joins the deep submucosal veins at the region about 2 cm below the gastro-oesophageal junction. These deep gastric submucosal veins directly connect with the oesophageal deep submucosal veins. These varices are almost always present with grade 3 or 4 oesophageal varices and not with small varices [59]. While none of the patients with IGV1 had oesophageal varices, about 50% of patients with GOV2 had associated large oesophageal varices.

In *segmental portal hypertension*, GV develop through the short and posterior gastric veins in the absence of oesophageal varices. Isolated GV could also develop in generalized portal hypertension due to cirrhosis or to non-cirrhotic portal hypertension.

MANAGEMENT OF GASTRIC VARICES

The management of GV is predominantly the management of bleeding from these lesions. The rationale and the methods for controlling the GV bleeding at present are empirical and far from satisfactory. Except for a subset of patients with persisting GOV1, there is little role for prophylactic therapy for GV.

The various treatment modalities employed for the control of gastric variceal bleeding are shown in Table 6 and include the following.

1   *Balloon tamponade.* With either the Linton–Nachlas tube or Sengstaken–Blakemore tube, primary haemostasis can be achieved in 30–80% of patients. The rebleeding rates are, however, high.

2   *Pharmacotherapy.* Only anecdotal unpublished data (Table 6) are available on the role of somatostatin and glypressin in the control of acute bleeding.

3   *Gastric variceal sclerotherapy (GVS).*

(a) *Agents:* a potent sclerosant with properties of instantaneous throm-bosis of the blood, with minimum tissue necrosis and negligible flow to the portal vein would be ideal for sclerotherapy of GV. Sodium tetradecyl sulphate [60], absolute alcohol [61], ethanolamine oleate [62] and a glue, butyl cyanoacrylate [46,63] have all been used successfully by different workers.

Table 6 Modalities to control acute gastric variceal bleeding.

| Modality | Success rate (%) | | |
	D'Amico et al.*	Calés et al.*	Sarin et al.*
Sclerotherapy	50	40	88
Drugs	70	50	—
Balloon tamponade	80	80	60
EVL	—	80	—
Glue	—	80	—
TIPS	—	90	67

EVL, endoscopic variceal ectasia; TIPS, transjugular intrahepatic portosystemic shunt.
* Unpublished observations.

(b) *Technique of GVS:* this could be done using either straight end-on technique for lesser curve variances (GOV1) or by retroflexion for fundal varices. Different modes of injection including paravariceal, intravariceal or a combination of the two methods have been employed for GV.

(c) *Emergency GVS:* the procedure is technically difficult in bleeding fundal varices, as the gushing blood makes visualization of the bleeding varix difficult. Trudeau and Prindiville [60] were able successfully to control GV bleeding in all nine of their patients; eight of the nine patients re-bled. With increasing expertise, good success in emergency control has now been reported by several workers, including ourselves (Table 7).

4 *Gastric variceal obturation.* This technique has been initiated by Gotlib *et al.* in 1981 [64]. Adhesive glues, namely isobutyl 2-cyanoacrylate (Bucrylate)

Table 7 Results of emergency gastric variceal sclerotherapy.

Reference	Agent	No. of patients actively bleeding	Success rate n (%)	Rebleed rate (%)
Bretagne et al. [50]	Polidocanol	10	6 (60)	63
Trudeau and Prindiville et al. [60]	STD	9	9 (100)	89
Ramond et al., [46]	Bucrylate	6	6 (100)	33
Sarin et al.,†	Absolute alcohol	16	14 (88)	19
Battaglia et al.,†	Bucrylate	23	18 (78)	22*

STD, sodium tetradecylsulphate.
* Five patients died.
† Unpublished data.

or n-butyl cyanoacrylate (Histoacryl) have been used for obturation of oesophagogastric varices. The glue is mixed with Lipiodol which makes the mixture radio-opaque and lengthens the butyl cyanoacrylate polymerization time. Success in the control of acute bleeds has been reported in 60–90% patients (Table 7). The rebleeding rates are, however, high.

5   *Transjugular intrahepatic portosystemic shunt.* TIPS may be life-saving in patients with massively bleeding GV who are poor risks for surgery. In one study, nine of 12 patients in whom TIPS was performed survived for 211 days on average [66]. In our own experience, TIPS was successful in controlling GV bleeding in three patients.

ELECTIVE THERAPY FOR GASTRIC VARICES

Drug therapy

There is limited information on the successful use of vasoactive agents in the treatment of GV.

Gastric variceal sclerotherapy

Repeated GVS has been used to obliterate GV (Table 8). Obliteration of GOV1 is often possible with a single session of GVS and was achieved in 16 of our 20 patients. Hosking and Johnson [39] also treated 24 of their patients with lesser curve varices by injection sclerotherapy at the squamocolumnar junction. This treatment is effective even if the blood flow is cephalad. Korula *et al.* [51] also observed successful obliteration of these varices with a single injection. Fundal varices (GOV2 and IGV1) generally require three or more sclerotherapy sessions. Trudeau and Prindiville [60] were not able to achieve obliteration of gastric varices despite five or six injection courses. They observed a high incidence of rebleeding which could partly be due to a rather

Table 8 Results of elective gastric variceal sclerotherapy.

Reference	No. of patients	Successful obliteration n (%)	rebleeding (n)
Yassin *et al.**	35	6	8
Ramond *et al.* [46]	27	19 (70)	6
Sarin *et al.*†	52	37 (71)	11#
Battaglia *et al.*†	51	30 (59)	13#

* Personal communication.
† Unpublished observations.

slow and incomplete obliteration achieved by 1.5% tetradecylsulphate. Using absolute alcohol, we were able to achieve obliteration in 25 (68%) of 37 patients with a mean of three sessions per patient [65]. Of the 12 remaining patients, obliteration could not be achieved in two, rebleeding occurred in 10. Six of the latter patients had fundal (GOV2, $n = 4$; IGV1, $n = 2$) varices.

Complications of gastric variceal sclerotherapy

Besides rebleeding, the most common complication of GVS is gastric mucosal ulcerations. Occasionally, these could be the site of rebleeding. In our experience, while sucralfate is of little value in oesophageal variceal ulcers, it is effective in accelerating the healing of gastric variceal ulcers. Although theoretically there is reasonable apprehension of splenic or portal vein thrombosis occurring after GVS, this complication has been rarely documented.

Gastric variceal obturation

The use of a glue appears to be effective (Tables 7 and 9) and particularly useful in treating GV since the incidence of post-sclerotherapy ulcers is quite low. Since bucrylate is not a sclerosant and does not cause thrombosis, obturation could be incomplete resulting in rebleeding. It remains to be seen whether addition of a sclerosant could improve the efficacy of glue injection. A comparison of glue injection and GVS has been recently reported and is shown in Table 9. In summary, GVS or obturation is effective in: (i) controlling acute gastric variceal bleeding; (ii) obliterating GOV1 and GOV2 in the majority of patients; (iii) success in treating IGV1 is limited due to rebleeding; and (iv) prophylactic sclerotherapy of GOV1 is safe and can be recommended.

Table 9 Comparison of histoacryl (HC) injection with ethanolamine oleate (EO) or absolute alcohol (AA).

Reference	Agent	No. of patients	Control of acute bleed n	(%)	Rebleeding n	(%)	Survival n	(%)
Oho et al. [62]	EO	24	16	(67)	8	(33)	16	(67)
	HC	23	22	(96)	8	(35)	12	(52)
Sarin et al. [00]	AA	7	5	(71)	3	(43)	6	(86)
	HC	7	6	(86)	3	(43)	6	(86)

SURGERY FOR GASTRIC VARICEAL BLEEDING

This section could be divided into management of GV due to: (i) segmental portal hypertension without any liver disease; and (ii) generalized portal hypertension.

Surgical treatment of segmental portal hypertension

Splenectomy effectively cures most patients with segmental portal hypertension without liver disease. Madsen *et al.* [45] reviewed the literature and described the course of 72 patients, 0 months to 24 years after splenectomy for segmental portal hypertension. Only two patients re-bled after splenectomy. Mortality after splenectomy has been reported to be around 7% [67].

Generalized portal hypertension

There is abundant information available on the surgical management of gastro-oesophageal varices. Little, however, is mentioned specifically about the management of gastric varices. There are no clear guidelines available on the selection of patients for a given surgical procedure. For patients with generalized portal hypertension and isolated GV, a definitive treatment is advisable. Hosking and Johnson [19] advocate variceal ligation with gastric devascularization for the control of active bleeding from such varices. However, if lesser-curve varices are associated, a shunt procedure may be better according to them. Alternatively, for patients with acute gastric variceal bleeding, an emergency shunt could be equally effective. According to Wood *et al.* [68] the shunt of choice is a large-bore H-graft mesocaval or mesorenal shunt. This shunt effectively controls the acute bleeding, is relatively simple to perform, does not impact on the subsequent transplant, and can be ligated after the transplant is completed.

ORTHOTOPIC LIVER TRANSPLANTATION (OLT)

The survival rates in transplanted patients [69] project OLT as a useful alternative to other modalities of treating GV. The differences become more prominent when the survival rates of Child's class C patients who received liver transplants (79% at 1 year and 71% at 5 years) are compared with those of Child's C patients who were treated with shunts (30–70% 1-year and 15-35% 5-year survival rats) [69]. These results of OLT bring a ray of hope for the large number of patients with cirrhosis and portal hypertension, including those with gastric varices. At present however, for a significant proportion of patients, transplant remains an expensive and difficult option, especially in the developing countries.

Acknowledgements

The kind assistance of Dr Felice Cosentino (Plates 1–6) and Dr Giorgio Battaglia (Plates 7–10) in providing the endoscopic photographs is greatly appreciated.

REFERENCES

1 McCormack TT, Sims J, Eyre-Brook I et al. Gastric lesions in portal hypertension: inflammatory gastritis or congestive gastropathy? Gut 1985, 26: 1226–1232.
2 Papazian A, Braillon A, Dupas JL, Sevenet F, Capron JP. Portal hypertensive gastric mucosa: an endoscopic study. Gut 1986; 27: 1199–1203.
3 Spina GP, Arcidiacono R, Bosch J et al. Gastric endoscopic features in portal hypertension: final report of a consensus conference. J Hepatol 1994; 21: 461–467.
4 Corbishley CM, Saverymuttu SH, Maxwell JD. Use of endoscopic biopsy for diagnosing congestive gastropathy. J Clin Pathol 1988; 41: 1187–1190.
5 Triger DR. Recognition of portal hypertensive gastropathy (PHG). In: Spina GP, Arcidiacono R (eds), Gastric Endoscopic Features in Portal Hypertension. Milan: Masson, 1994: 13–17.
6 Sarin SK, Sreniwas DV, Lahoti D, Saraya A. Factors influencing development of congestive gastropathy in patients with portal hypertension. Gastroenterology 1992; 102: 994–999.
7 Calés P, Zabotto B, Meskens C et al. Gastric endoscopic features in cirrhosis. Observer variability, interassociations and relationship to hepatic dysfunction. Gastroenterology 1990; 98: 156–162.
8 Sarin SK, Misra SP, Singal AK, Thorat V, Broor SL. Evaluation of the incidence and significance of mosaic pattern in patients with cirrhosis, noncirrhotic portal fibrosis and extrahepatic obstruction. Am J Gastroenterol 1988; 83: 1235–1239.
9 Misra SP, Dwivedi M, Misra V et al. Endoscopic and histologic appearance of the gastric mucosa in patients with portal hypertension. Gastrointest Endosc 1990; 36: 575–579.
10 Perez Ayuso RM, Pique JM, Bosch et al. Propranolol in the prevention of rebleeding from portal hypertensive gastropathy. Lancet 1991; 337: 1431–1434.
11 Jabbari M, Cherry R, Lough JO, Daly DS, Innear DG, Gorski CA. Gastric antral vascular ectasia: the watermelon stomach. Gastroenterology 1984; 87: 1165–1170.
12 Gostout CJ, Viggiano TR, Ahlquist DA et al. The clinical and endoscopic spectrum of the watermelon stomach. J Clin Gastroenterol 1992; 15: 256–263.
13 Payen JL, Calés P, Voigt JJ et al.. Severe portal hypertensive gastropathy and antral vascular ectasia are distinct entities in patients with cirrhosis. Gastroenterology 1995; 108: 138–144.
14 Ohta M, Hashizume M, Higashi H et al. Portal and gastric mucosal hemodynamics in cirrhotic patients with portal-hypertensive gastropathy. Hepatology 1994; 20: 1432–1436.

15 D'Amico G, Montalbano L, Traina M *et al*. Natural history of congestive gastropathy in cirrhosis. *Gastroenterology* 1990; **9**: 1558–1564.

16 Hon MC, Lin HC, Chen CH *et al*. Change of portal hypertensive gastropathy following EVL or sclerotherapy. *Hepatology* 1994; **20**: 104A.

17 Sarin SK, Govil A, Jain AK *et al*. Prospective randomized trial of endoscopic sclerotherapy versus variceal band ligation for bleeding esophageal varices: influence on gastropathy, gastric varices and variceal recurrence (abstract). *Gastroenterology* 1995; **108**: A1163.

18 Sarin SK. Non-cirrhotic portal fibrosis. *Gut* 1989; **30**: 406–415.

19 Sarfeh IJ, Tarnawski A, Malki A, Mason GR, Mach T, Ivery KJ. Portal hypertension and gastric mucosal injury in rats. *Gastroenterology* 1993; **84**: 987–993.

20 Sarfeh IJ, Tarnawski A, Maeda R *et al*. The gastric mucosa in portal hypertension. Effect of topical bile acid. *Scand J Gastroenterol* 1984; **19** (Suppl. 92): 189–194.

21 Quintero E, Pique JP, Bombi JA *et al*. Gastric mucosal vascular ectasias causing bleeding in cirrhosis. *Gastroenterology* 1987; **93**: 1054–1061.

22 Iwao T, Toyonaga A, Sumino M *et al*. Portal hypertensive gastropathy in patients with cirrhosis. *Gastroenterology* 1992; **102**: 2060–2065.

23 Iweao T, Toyanaga A, Ikegami M *et al*. Reduced gastric mucosal blood flow in patients with portal-hypertensive gastropathy. *Hepatology* 1993; **18**: 36–40.

24 Groszmann RJ, Colombato LA. Gastric vascular changes in portal hypertension. *Hepatology* 1988; **8**: 1708–1710.

25 Piqué JM, Pizcueta MP, Perez RM, Bosch J. Effects of propranolol on gastric mucosal blood flow and acid secretion in portal hypertensive rats. *Hepatology* 1990; **12**: 476–480.

26 Panés J, Bordas J, Piqué J *et al*. Increased gastric mucosal perfusion in cirrhotic patients with portal hypertensive gastropathy. *Gastroenterology* 1992; **103**: 1875–1882.

27 Panés J, Bordas JM, Piqué JP *et al*. Effects of propranolol on gastric mucosal perfusion in cirrhotic patients with portal hypertensive gastropathy. *Hepatology* 1992; **17**: 213–218.

28 Foster PN, Wyatt JI, Bullimore DW, Losowsky MS. Gastric mucosa in patients with portal hypertension: prevalence of capillary dilatation and *Campylobacter pylori*. *J Clin Pathol* 1989; **42**: 919–921.

29 Lam SK. Hypergastrinemia in cirrhosis of the liver. *Gut* 1976; **17**: 700–708.

30 Gaur SK, Vij JC, Sarin SK, Anand BS. Gastric secretory studies in cirrhosis and non-cirrhotic portal fibrosis. *Digestion* 1988; **39**: 151–155.

31 Lamarque D, Levoir D, Duvoux C *et al*. Measurement of gastric intramucosal pH in patients with cirrhosis and portal hypertensive gastropathy. *Gastroenterol Clin Biol* 1994; **18**: 969–74.

32 Ganguly S, Sarin SK, Bhatia V, Lahoti D. The prevalence and spectrum of colonic lesions in patients with cirrhosis and noncirrhotic portal hypertension. *Hepatology* 1995; **21**: 1226–1231.

33 Eleftheriadis E, Kotzampassi K, Aletras H. The influence of sclerotherapy on gastric mucosal blood flow distribution. *Am Surg* 1990; **56**: 593–593.

34 Hosking SW, Kennedy HJ, Seddon I *et al*. The role of propranolol in congestive gastropathy of portal hypertension. *Hepatology* 1987; **7**: 437–441.

35 Van Cutsem E, Rutgeerts P, Vantrappen G. Treatment of bleeding gastrointestinal vascular malformations with oestrogen–progesterone. *Lancet* 1990; **335**: 953–955.

36 Panés J, Casadevall M, Fernandez M *et al*. Gastric microcirculatory changes of portal-hypertensive rats can be attenuated by long-term estrogen–progestagen treatment.

Hepatology 1994; **20**: 1261–1270.

37 Evans JA, Delany F. Gastric varices. *Radiology* 1953; **60**: 46–52.

38 Karr S, Wohl GT. Clinical importance of gastric varices. *N Engl J Med* 1960; **263**: 665–669.

39 Hosking SW, Johnson AG. Gastric varices: a proposed classification to management. *Br J Surg* 1988; **75**: 195–196.

40 Watanabe K, Kimura K, Matsutani S *et al.* Portal hemodynamics in patients with gastric varices. A study in 230 patients with oesophageal or gastric varices using portal vein catheterization. *Gastroenterology* 1988; **95**, 434–440.

41 Sarin SK, Lahoti D, Saxena SP, Murthi NS, Makwane UK. Prevalence, classification and natural history of gastric varices: long term follow-up study in 568 patients with portal hypertension. *Hepatology* 1992; **16**: 1343–1349.

42 Battaglia G, Gerunda G. NIEC classification of gastric varices. In: Spina GP, Arcidiacono R (eds), *Gastric Endoscopic Features in Portal Hypertension*. Milan: Masson, 1994: 69–72.

43 Caletti G, Brocchi E, Baraldini M *et al.* Assessment of portal hypertension by endoscopic ultrasonography. *Gastrointest Endosc* 1990; **36**: S21–S27.

44 Hashizume M, Kitano S, Yamaga H *et al.* Endoscopic classification of gastric varices. *Gastrointest Endosc* 1990; **36**: 276–280.

45 Madsen MS, Petersen TH, Sommer H. Segmental portal hypertension. *Ann Surg* 1986; **204**: 72–77.

46 Ramond MJ, Valla D, Mosnier JF *et al.* Successful endoscopic obliteration of gastric varices with butyl cyanoacrylate. *Hepatology* 1989; **10**: 488–493.

47 Terés J, Cecilia A, Bordas JM *et al.* Oesophageal tamponade for bleeding varices. Controlled trial between the Sengstaken Blakemore tube and the Linton Nachlas tube. *Gastroenterology* 1978; **75**: 566–569.

48 Paquet KJ. Open discussion on technical aspects of injection sclerotherapy. In: Westaby D, McDougall BRD, Williams R (eds), *Variceal Bleeding*. London: Pitman Press, 1982: 215–217.

49 Weissberg J, Stein DT, Fogel M, Knauer CM, Gregory PB. Variceal bleeding. Does it matter to the patient whether his gastric or oesophageal varices bleed? *Gastroenterology* 1984; **86**: 1296 (Abstract).

50 Bretagne JF, Dudicourt JC, Morisot D *et al.* Is endoscopic variceal sclerotherapy effective for the treatment of gastric varices? *Dig Dis Sci* 1986; **31**: A505S.

51 Korula J, Chin K, Ko Y, Yamada S. Demonstration of two distinct subsets of gastric varices: observations during a seven year study of endoscopic sclerotherapy. *Dig Dis Sci* 1991; **36**: 303–309.

52 Little AG, Moosa AR. Gastrointestinal hemorrhage from left sided portal hypertension; an unappreciated complication of pancreatitis. *Am J Surg* 1981; **141**: 153–158.

53 Mathur SK, Dalvi AN, Someshwar V, Supe AN, Ramakhantan R. Endoscopic and radiological appraisal of gastric varices. *Br J Surg* 1990; **77**: 432–5.

54 Hedberg CE, Fowler DL, Ryan RLR. Injection sclerotherapy of oesophageal varices using ethanolamine oleate. *Am J Surg* 1987; **143**: 426–431.

55 Takase Y, Ozak A, Orii R *et al.* Injection sclerotherapy of oesophageal varices for patients undergoing emergency and elective surgery. *Surgery* 1982; **92**: 474–479.

56 Jorge AD, Adam J, Seittert L, Segal E. Sclerotherapy of oesophageal varices – an Argentinian experience. *Endoscopy* 1983; **15**: 141–143.

57 Schubert TT, Schnell GA, Walden JM. Bleeding from varices in the gastric fundus complicating sclerotherapy. *Gastrointest Endosc* 1989; **35**: 268–269.

58 Sarin SK, Nundy S. Subclinical encephalopathy after postasystemic shunts in patients with non-cirrhotic portal fibrosis. *Liver* 1985; **5**: 142–146.

59 Sarin SK, Kumar A. Gastric varices: profile, classification and management. *Am J Gastroenterol* 1989; **84**: 1244–1249.

60 Trudeau W, Prindiville T. Endoscopic injection sclerosis in bleeding gastric varices. *Gastrointest Endosc* 1985; **32**: 264–268.

61 Sarin SK, Sachdev G, Nanda R *et al.* Endoscopic sclerotherapy in the treatment of gastric varices. *Br J Surg* 1988; **75**: 747–750.

62 Oho K, Toyonaga A, Iwao T *et al.* Sclerotherapy for bleeding gastric varices: ethanolamine oleate versus butyl-cyanoacrylate. *Hepatology* 1994; **20**: A107.

63 Soehendra N, Nam VC, Grimm H *et al.* Endoscopic obliteration of large esophagogastric varices with Bucrylate. *Endoscopy* 1986; **18**: 25–26.

64 Gotlib JP, Demma I, Fonsecca A *et al.* Resultats a 1 an du traitement endoscopique electif des hemorragies par rupture de varices oesophagiennes chez le cirrhotique (abstract). *Gastroenterol Clin Biol* 1984; **8**: 133A.

65 Sarin SK, Lahoti D. Management of gastric varices. *Baillière's Clin Gastroenterol* 1992; **6**: 527–548.

66 Kuradusenge P, Russeau H, Vinel JP *et al.* Traitement des hemorragies par rupture de varices cardio-tuberositaires par anastomose porto-systemique intrahepatique par voie transjugulaire. *Gastroenterol Clin Biol* 1993; **17**: 431–434.

67 Toder O Chr. Splenic vein thrombosis with bleeding gastrooesophageal varices. Report of 2 splenectomized cases and review of the literature. *Acta Chir Scand* 1984; **150**: 265–268.

68 Wood RP, Shaw BW Jr, Rikkers LF. Liver transplantation for variceal hemorrhage. *Surg Clin N Am* 1990; **70**: 449–461.

69 Iwatsuki S, Starzl TE, Todo S *et al.* Liver transplantation in the treatment of bleeding oesophageal varices. *Surgery* 1987; **104**: 697–701.

Baveno II Consensus Statements:
Portal Hypertensive Gastropathy and Gastric Varices

Shiv K. Sarin (Chairman), Giorgio Battaglia, Paul Calés, Lorenzo Cestari, Giorgio Gerunda and Massimo Primignani

Portal hypertensive gastropathy

1   For the diagnosis of acute GI bleed due to PHG we need:
   - Endoscopic evidence of active bleeding lesion (after washing or removing clots, full distension)
   - If GV/oesophageal varices present, repeat endoscopy within 12–24 hours.

2   We should use an objective scoring system: 'PHG/mucosal lesional score'. It gives opportunity to evaluate PHG. More data are required about GAVE.

3   Criteria for assessing chronic bleeding:
   - Faecal blood loss
   - ≥ 2 g/dl drop in Hb in 3 months
   - Low transferrin saturation

4   Chronic bleed due to PHG should be accepted only if:
   - Endoscopic lesions are present
   - Colopathy/duodenopathy are absent
   - Bone marrow suppression is absent, no associated renal disease and no NSAIDs.

Gastric varices

1   We propose the NIEC classification for GV.
2   Diagnostic modalities:
   - Endoscopy/two observers needed to confirm
   - Endosonography – needs further evaluation.
3   Indications for GV treatment:
   - Bleeding GV
   - History of GV bleed
   - Prophylactic – needs further evaluation.
4   Treatment options and protocol:
   - Emergency – available options need evaluation by controlled trials
   - Elective – available options need evaluation by controlled trials.

Imaging Techniques and Haemodynamic Measurements in Portal Hypertension

Luigi Bolondi, Fabio Piscaglia, Sebastiano Siringo,
Stefano Gaiani and Gianni Zironi

INTRODUCTION

Over the past few years, the development and increasing clinical use of non-invasive techniques, which allow imaging of the portal venous system and its abnormalities and the performance of haemodynamic measurements, have progressively reduced the utilization of invasive techniques such as angiography, used largely in the past. This latter method, however, still remains the 'gold standard' for preoperative imaging of the portal venous system in the few patients who are candidates for surgical portosystemic anastomosis [1]. While real-time ultrasound (US) and particularly the duplex and colour Doppler methods are now increasingly employed for the study of portal hypertensive patients, the use of computed tomography (CT) in this field, even with the most recent technical developments, such as the spiral method [2], has never gained much popularity. Other recently developed non-invasive methods which can provide a morphological assessment of portal hypertension, together with haemodynamic information, are magnetic resonance (MR) angiography and per-rectal scintigraphy. Their use, how-ever, is still limited because of the scarce availability of MR and nuclear medicine resources and the lack of demonstration of the clinical usefulness and advantages of these methods over real-time US and colour Doppler. Other, more invasive techniques, such as endoscopic ultrasonography (EUs) and the endoscopic measurement of variceal pressure through a pressure-sensitive gauge, are increasingly used, but their diagnostic and prognostic value remain to be defined. Portal pressure is the most important haemo-dynamic parameter, but the indications for its use in clinical practice are controversial. It can be obtained by catheterization of the hepatic vein, or percutaneously by puncture of an intrahepatic branch of the portal vein. The latter technique, however, has been scarcely used in the past few years because of its invasiveness, and measurement of hepatic venous pressure gradient through catheterization of the hepatic veins remains the most used method to assess pressure in the portal venous system. We shall provide an overview of the most recent advances and of the impact of these techniques in the clinical assessment of portal hypertensive patients.

DOPPLER ULTRASOUND FLOWMETRY

Clinical applications of Doppler flowmetry of hepatic vessels include the assessment of the presence, direction and characteristics of blood flow. The quantitative measurement of the volume of blood flow has also been attempted in some major abdominal arteries and veins, and this possibility is awakening increasing interest. The presence of blood flow within the portal vein is the simplest Doppler finding to ascertain. The diagnosis of portal vein obstruction is sometimes uncertain in real-time US imaging, especially in cases of recent thrombosis, when the echo pattern of the thrombus is markedly hypoechoic and may be missed, so that the lumen appears patent. In these cases the absence of the Doppler signal from the portal vein confirms the diagnosis. In other instances the finding of the Doppler signal can contribute to distinguishing a partial thrombosis from a complete obstruction, where no signal can be detected at the porta hepatis. For this purpose Doppler flowmetry may be even more accurate than arterioportography, which can suggest erroneously a portal thrombosis in the case of complete diversion of the contrast medium into large portosystemic collaterals. The extensive application of Doppler US flowmetry in non-selected patients affected by liver cirrhosis contributed to clarifying the prevalence of partial and complete portal thrombosis, which have recently been estimated at 5.7 and 1.8%, respectively [3]. Pulsed Doppler and colour flow mapping may also be helpful in identifying flow in the collateral vessels, which often develops as a consequence of portal hypertension.

Direction of blood flow is another unequivocal qualitative finding provided by Doppler US. Its importance in the investigation of hepatic haemodynamics is striking. There are conflicting data regarding the prevalence of a reversed flow in the major vessels of the portal venous system in liver cirrhosis; in our series it was 8.3% [3]. Reversal of flow is often related to the presence of large portosystemic collaterals such as splenorenal shunts. A significantly higher rate of bleeding was demonstrated in patients with hepatopetal flow, thus suggesting a protective role of reversed flow against the risk of variceal bleeding.

One of the most striking characteristics of the systemic haemodynamics of cirrhotic patients is the hyperdynamic circulation associated with a fall in arterial resistance. This phenomenon has been studied using the Doppler method, which showed that the pulsatility index (an indirect measurement of arterial impedance, calculated as systolic–diastolic flow velocity difference divided by mean flow velocity) of the superior mesenteric artery is significantly decreased in patients with liver cirrhosis [4]. Analysis of the Doppler signals arising from hepatic veins may also provide interesting data. The hepatic veins in healthy humans display a triphasic waveform depending upon cardiac cycle and particularly the fluctuating right atrial pressure. These phasic variations of flow are completely lost in 18.3% of cases of liver cirrhosis with portal hypertension and greatly reduced in another 31.7% [5]. The pathophysiology of this behaviour is unclear. A significant correlation ($P < 0.01$) has been found with the decrease in the resistance index in the superior mesenteric artery and the increase in the Child–Pugh score. These data suggest that the hyperdynamic circulation and the severity of the liver tissue alterations could play a role in determining changes in the hepatic vein waveform. Absence, reversal or steady flow in the hepatic veins may be consistent with the diagnosis of Budd–Chiari syndrome [6].

Quantitative haemodynamic measurements, such as that of portal vein blood flow volume, have always proved difficult. Electromagnetic flow-metry, indocyanine green clearance, indicator dilution and thermodilution techniques do not completely satisfy the clinical need. Non-invasive measurements using Doppler US have therefore attracted a great deal of attention in recent years. Possible sources of errors in the quantitative esti-mates of blood flow in the portal vein have been outlined by Gill [7] and reconsidered by Burns [8] and Dauzat and Pomier-Layrargues [9]. The reproducibility of Doppler measurements has attracted the interest of investigators and is certainly important for the clinical application of the quantitative Doppler parameters. Previous studies [10,11] have demon-strated a significant inter- and intra-observer variability for portal flow and velocity calculation. Causes for inadequate reproducibility have been iden-tified as: (i) differing observer experience; (ii) non-standardized techniques of examination; (iii) inclusion of subjects unsuitable for the examination; and (iv) actual variation of the parameters measured [12]. A more recent study [13] has shown that a cooperative training of the operators can significantly reduce the interobserver variability in quantitative measurements. Instru-mentation variability [13] has also been ascertained, thus suggesting that follow-up examinations must be carried out on the same equipment and with the same transducer and angle. At present, it is reasonable to suppose that the Doppler spectrum reflects the actual blood flow in the portal vein, although the absolute values expressed in terms of millimetres per minute may not correspond to the real flow volume. The validity of the assessment of changes in mean velocity and flow volume by Doppler flowmetry in the same subject under different conditions is unanimously accepted [14], since possible sources of error in measuring absolute values are expected to affect different measurements in the same way. The method therefore seems suitable for *in vivo* monitoring of acute haemodynamic changes in the portal vein such as those induced by food [15], hormones [16], drugs and other vasoactive substances, as well as circadian variations of portal flow [17]. Quantitative measurements of flow in the portal vein demonstrated that the velocity is reduced, to a greater or lesser degree, in cirrhotic patients in comparison with healthy subjects [18]. Large splenorenal collaterals may reduce portal flow and even cause its reversal while a patent and dilated para-umbilical vein may explain high velocity and volume of portal flow. As far as the clinical meaning of these collaterals is concerned, Mostbeck *et al.* [19] reported that a massive hepatofugal flow through a large para-umbilical vein may reduce the risk of variceal bleeding.

Duplex Doppler has also been recently used to ascertain the presence of an increased renal vascular resistance [20,21] by assessing the resistance index of the intraparenchymal renal arteries. High intrarenal vascular resistances have been found both in the pre-ascitic and ascitic stages of the disease. Diuretic treatment further increases resistances [21]. A significant correlation with the severity of liver disease, with increasing values of resistance index in patients with higher Child–Pugh scores, has also been demonstrated [22]. Finally, the intrarenal resistance index has been proposed as a significant prognostic factor for survival [23].

Doppler flowmetry may also be useful in understanding the mechanism of the effect of drugs on the portal venous system, in detecting non-responders and in establishing the dosage and efficacy of new drugs [24,25]. Furthermore, the effect of a drug on collateral circulation, and particularly in the left gastric vein, can be investigated in selected patients with large and straight collaterals [26].

A recent study disclosed a new clinical contribution of Doppler US flowmetry, particularly of portal vein diameter and flow velocity, when added to clinical, biochemical and endoscopic parameters. It has been demonstrated that these parameters improve the prediction of bleeding [27]. Other previous studies had already shown the prognostic value of portal vein velocity in predicting death [28] and its correlation with the most important functional and endoscopic parameters [29].

MAGNETIC RESONANCE ANGIOGRAPHY

Since its first introduction in clinical practice, MR imaging has been used to evaluate the patency of portal vessels, but a number of attempts have also been made to measure the blood flow velocity. The possibility of measuring the velocity of a fluid by MR has been known since the late 1980s [30]. Different techniques, such as direct bolus imaging (DBI) [30,31] and quantitative phase-contrast [32,33] have been employed. Both methods require breath-holding for at least 12 seconds and provide information regarding flow direction and velocity and consequently, by measuring the cross-sectional area of the vessel, flow volume. Portosystemic collaterals can be easily identified [31] and reversed portal blood flow can be shown. A close correlation with measurements obtained by pulsed Doppler has been obtained [30,33] and the reduction of flow velocity in the portal vein has been confirmed in cirrhotic patients [33]. Acute changes in flow velocity, determined by various stimuli (ethanol, glucose administration), can be assessed by MR angiography [30]. Theoretical advantages of this technique over Doppler US are that it is independent of the operator, is not limited by obesity and does not need a correction for the angle of insonation. Flow measurement in the main portal vein by cine-phase-contrast MR imaging has been correlated with the presence of variceal haemorrhage within 2 years [32]; a significant association was found between variceal haemorrhage and high portal venous flow. This finding provides a further insight into the pathophysiology of portal hypertension and particularly in the balance between increased intrahepatic resistance and hyperdynamic splanchnic flow.

ENDOSCOPIC ULTRASOUND

Endoscopic US provides various information about both the morphology and haemodynamics of the azygos vein and peri-oesophageal collaterals of portal hypertensive patients. Morphological imaging is performed by rotating probes providing a 360° image. In clinical practice this technique is used in portal hypertensive patients to detect the presence and size of peri-oesophageal collateral vessels, size of the azygos vein and presence of gastric fundic varices, whose differentiation from normal gastric rugae or polyps is more precise than by conventional diagnostic endoscopy. So far, routine endoscopy is much more sensitive and precise than endoscopic US in the detection of oesophageal varices and of portal hypertensive gastropathy (PHG) [34]. The calibre of the azygos vein, measured at endoscopic US, has proved significantly larger in cirrhotic patients compared with that in controls [34]. The prognostic role of this technique to assess the risk of bleeding and its usefulness in following the outcome of endoscopic sclerotherapy has not been established. The use of an endoscopic convex probe connected to an instrumentation provided with Doppler facilities allows the assessment of blood flow velocity – and consequently blood flow volume – in the azygos vein [35]. Until now, this technique still requires some further standardization and its use is limited to research protocols. A possible field of application could be the monitoring of acute (upon pharmacological treatment) haemodynamic changes in the azygos vein, which may be different from those present in the portal trunk.

VARICEAL PRESSURE MEASUREMENTS

Variceal pressure can be measured by different techniques performed during operative endoscopy. Some techniques are considered invasive, since variceal pressure is directly measured by a needle puncture of the varix itself, while some others use non-invasive methods such as the application of a pressure-sensitive gauge to the varix. This type of measurement has raised much interest since the 1980s as some workers reported a higher incidence of bleeding in patients with high variceal pressure [36] and showed correlations between variceal pressure and other parameters predictive of oesophageal bleeding (variceal size, presence of red signs, degree of liver dysfunction, portal blood flow velocity and previous variceal bleeding episodes) [36–39]. However, the real predictive value of variceal pressure has not been clarified so far and clinical prospective trials are still awaited. More recently, some studies used variceal pressure together with other haemodynamic and endoscopic data to investigate further the development of portal hypertensive gastropathy [40,41]. This technique has recently been used to investigate directly the acute and chronic effects of different drugs and of portosystemic surgical shunts on variceal pressure [42–47].

MEASUREMENTS OF AZYGOS BLOOD FLOW

Azygos blood flow measurement is performed by a local continuous thermodilution method. In patients with portal hypertension it correlates neither with the presence and size of oesophageal varices nor with the risk of bleeding from ruptured varices [48], probably since this vessel drains not only blood from the oesophagus, but also from para-oesophageal and mediastinal vessels [49]. Measurements of azygos blood flow could be useful for monitoring rapid haemodynamic changes, as those determined by pharmacological treatment. In the past few years, however, no substantial new data have been derived with this method.

MEASUREMENTS OF HEPATIC VENOUS PRESSURE GRADIENT (HVPG)

This type of haemodynamic measurement has not undergone major technical improvement in the past years, since most studies on portal hypertension in the 1970s and 1980s already relied on this approach. In patients with cirrhosis, an elevated HVPG is present and correlates with the severity of liver disease estimated by the Child–Pugh classification. Although several studies reported a threshold level of 12 mmHg, below which variceal bleeding should virtually not occur [50], prospective studies showed that HVPG, measured only once at entry into the study, is not a good index of bleeding risk [49]. In one recent trial [51] of prophylactic sclerotherapy to prevent the first variceal bleeding, 32% of patients with HVPG < 12 mmHg bled and the addition of HVPG to variceal size was not a better criterion than variceal size alone to identify patients at higher risk of bleeding. In the past years, however, the application of this technique to new clinical protocols produced new evidence of its usefulness in portal hypertensive patients. Repeated measurements of HVPG permitted elucidation of haemodynamic events caused by drug treatment or by placebo in the prevention of first variceal haemorrhage [52], showing the efficacy of propranolol in reducing HVPG and consequently the incidence of bleeding episodes in the first year of treatment. This haemodynamic evaluation also showed the efficacy of nitrate monotherapy, or combined with beta-blockers, to reduce HVPG in long-term studies [53,54]. Continuous monitoring of HVPG proved safe and allowed, in patients with bleeding oesophageal varices [55], a reliable estimation of the role of portal pressure on the risk of continued bleeding or early rebleeding, reported to occur only as HVPG $\geqslant 16$ mmHg. Moreover, in another study on non-bleeding patients it showed the presence of circadian variations in portal pressure [56]. Finally, HVPG determined at entry was also reported to improve the accuracy of prognostic indexes for survival [57].

RADIONUCLIDE TECHNIQUES

The application of radionuclide techniques in portal hypertension is related to the detection and quantification of portosystemic shunting, expressed as shunt index (e.g. heart radioactivity/heart + liver radioactivity at scheduled time after administration) varying from 0 to 100%. Different radioactive compounds can be used, such as 99 m-technetium pertechnetate or 201-thallium or ^{123}I-iodoamphetamine. This latter compound can be administered either directly in duodenum or per os in enteric-coated capsules to detect superior mesenteric shunting, whereas all the compounds mentioned above can be administered per rectum, allowing detection of inferior mesenteric vein shunting, which is higher than the superior mesenteric vein shunt [58]. The shunt index is reported to be useful to differentiate non-invasively chronic hepatitis from cirrhosis [59], to correlate with the progression of the disease [58] and to improve prediction of poor prognosis [60]. Finally, quantitative sequential scintigraphy, which measures the portal contribution to liver perfusion and portosystemic shunting, has been reported to improve the overall sensitivity of endoscopy in detecting the presence of portal hypertension (from 66.7 to 86.1%) [61]. These techniques, however, are not currently applied in clinical practice and their use remains limited to research protocols.

REFERENCES

1 Okuda K, Takayasu K, Matsutani S. Angiography in portal hypertension. *Gastroenterol Clin N Am* 1992; **21**: 61–83.

2 Bluemke DA, Urban B, Fishman EK. Spiral CT of the liver: current applications. *Semin Ultrasound CT MR 1994;* **15**(2): 107–121.

3 Gaiani S, Bolondi L, Li Bassi L, Zironi G, Siringo S, Barbara L. Prevalence of spontaneous hepatofugal flow in liver cirrhosis. Clinical and endoscopical correlation in 228 patients. *Gastroenterology* 1991; **100**: 160–167.

4 Sabbà C, Ferraioli G, Genecin P *et al.* Evaluation of postprandial hyperemia in superior meseneric artery and portal vein in healthy and cirrhotic humans: an operator-blind echo-Doppler study. *Hepatology* 1991; **13**: 714–718.

5 Bolondi L, Li Bassi S, Gaiani S *et al.* Liver cirrhosis: changes of Doppler waveform of hepatic veins. *Radiology* 1991; **178**: 513–516.

6 Bolondi L, Gaiani S, Li Bassi S *et al.* Diagnosis of Budd–Chiari syndrome by pulsed Doppler ultrasound. *Gastroenterology* 1991; **100**: 1324–1329.

7 Gill RW. Measurement of blood flow by ultrasound: accuracy and sources of error. *Ultrasound Med Biol* 1985; **11**: 625–641.

8 Burns P. Doppler flowmetry and portal hypertension. *Gastroenterology* 1987; **92**: 824–826.

9 Dauzat M, Pomier-Layrargues G. Portal vein blood flow measurements using pulsed Doppler and electromagnetic flowmetry in dogs: a comparative study. *Gastroenterology* 1989; **96**: 913–919.

10 Sabbà C, Weltin G, Cicchetti DV *et al.* Observer variability in echo-Doppler measurements of portal flow in cirrhotic patients and normal volunteers. *Gastroenterology* 1990; **98**: 1603–1611.

11 DeVries PJ, Van Hattum J, Hoekstra JBL, De Hooge P. Duplex Doppler measurements of portal venous flow in normal subjects: inter- and intra-observer variability. *J Hepatol* 1991; **13**: 358–363.

12 Bolondi L, Gaiani S, Barbara L. Accuracy and reproducibility of portal flow measurement by Doppler US. *J Hepatol* 1991; **13**: 269–273.

13 Sabbà C, Merkel C, Zoli *et al.* Interobserver and interequipment variability of echo-Doppler examination of the portal vein: effect of a cooperative training program. *Hepatology* 1995; **21**: 428–433.

14 Barbara L. The value of Doppler US in the study of hepatic hemodynamics. Consensus conference, Bologna, 12 Sept 1989. *J Hepatol* 1990; **10**: 353–355.

15 Gaiani S, Bolondi L, Li Bassi S, Santi V, Zironi G, Barbara L. Effect of meal on portal hemodynamics in healthy humans and in patients with chronic liver disease. *Hepatology* 1989; **9**: 815–819.

16 Bolondi L, Gaiani S, Li Bassi S, Casanova P, Zironi G, Barbara L. Effect of secretin on portal venous flow. *Gut* 1990; **31**: 1306–1310.

17 Alvarez D, Golombek D, Lopez P *et al.* Diurnal fluctuations of portal and systemic hemodynamic parameters in patients with cirrhosis. *Hepatology* 1994; **20**: 1198–1203.

18 Zironi G, Gaiani S, Fenyves D *et al.* Value of measurement of mean portal flow velocity by Doppler flowmetry in the diagnosis of portal hypertension. *J Hepatol* 1992; **16**: 298–303.

19 Mostbeck GH, Wittich GR, Herold C *et al.* Hemodynamic significance of the paraumbilical vein in portal hypertension: assessment with duplex US. *Radiology* 1989; **170**: 339–342.

20 Platt JP, Marn CS, Baliga PK, Ellis J, Rubin JM, Merion RM. Renal dysfunction in hepatic disease: early identification with renal duplex Doppler US in patients who undergo liver transplantation. *Radiology* 1992; **183**: 801–806.

21 Sacerdoti D, Bolognesi M, Merkel C, Angeli P, Gatta A. Renal vasoconstriction in cirrhosis evaluated by duplex Doppler ultrasonography. *Hepatology* 1993; **17**: 219–224.

22 Zironi G, Bolondi L, Gaiani S, Sofia S, Siringo S, Barbara L. Relationship between changes of intrarenal arterial resistances and severity of liver cirrhosis: a Doppler US investigation. *Eur J Ultrasound* 1994; **1**: 51–57.

23 Maroto A, Ginès A, Salò J *et al.* Diagnosis of functional kidney failure of cirrhosis with Doppler sonography: prognostic value of resistive index. *Hepatology* 1994; **20**: 839–844.

24 Luca A, Garcia-Pagan JC, Feu F *et al.* Noninvasive measurement of femoral blood flow and portal pressure response to propranolol in patients with cirrhosis. *Hepatology* 1995; **21**: 83–88.

25 Merkel C, Sacerdoti D, Bolognesi M, Enzo E, Marin R, Gatta A. Failure of acute challenge with nadolol to predict long-term portal hemodynamic effect in patients with cirrhosis: an assessment using invasive and non-invasive techniques. *Ital J Gastroenter* 1994; **26**: 208 (Abstract).

26 Gaiani S, Bolondi L, Fenyves D, Zironi G, Rigamonti A, Barbara L. Effect of propranolol on portosystemic collateral circulation in patients with liver cirrhosis. *Hepatology* 1991; **14**: 824–829.

27 Siringo S, Bolondi L, Gaiani S *et al.* Timing of the first variceal hemorrhage in cirrhotic patients: prospective evaluation of Doppler flowmetry, endoscopy and clinical parameters. *Hepatology* 1994; **20**: 66–73.

28 Zoli M, Marchesini G, Brunori A, Cordiani MR, Pisi E. Portal venous flow in response to acute beta-blocker and vasodilatory treatment in patients with liver cirrhosis. *Hepatology* 1986; **6**: 1248–1251.

29 Siringo S, Bolondi L, Gaiani *et al.* The relationship of endoscopy, portal Doppler ultrasound flowmetry and clinical and biochemical tests in cirrhosis. *J Hepatol* 1994; **20**: 11–18.

30 Tamada T, Moriyasu F, Ono S *et al.* Portal blood flow: measurement with MR imaging. *Radiology* 1989; **173**: 639–644.

31 Edelman RR, Zhao B, Liu C *et al.* MR angiography and dynamic flow evaluation of the portal venous system. *AJR* 1989; **153**: 755–760.

32 Burkart DJ, Johnson CD, Ehman RL, Weaver AL, Ilstrup DM. Evaluation of portal venous hypertension with cine phase-contrast MR flow measurements: high association of hyperdynamic portal flow with variceal hemorrhage. *Radiology* 1993; **188**: 643–648.

33 Applegate GR, Thaete FL, Meyers SP *et al.* Blood flow in the portal vein: velocity quantitation with phase-contrast MR angiography. *Radiology* 1993; **187**: 253–256.

34 Caletti GC, Brocchi E, Baraldini M, Ferrari A, Gibilaro M, Barbara L. Assessment of portal hypertension by endoscopic ultrasonography. *Gastrointest Endosc* 1990; **36**: S21–27.

35 Bolondi L, Gaiani S, Zironi G, Fornari F, Siringo S, Barbara L. Color Doppler endosonography in the study of portal hypertension. In Heyder N, Hahn EG, Goldberg BB (eds) *Innovations in Abdominal Ultrasound*. Heidelberg: Springer-Verlag, 1992: 61–69.

36 Rigau J, Bosch J, Bordas J *et al.* Endoscopic measurement of variceal pressure in cir-

rhosis: correlation with portal pressure and variceal hemorrhage. *Gastroenterology* 1989; **96**: 873–880.

37 Staritz M, Poralla T, Meyer zum Buschenfelde KH. Intravascular esophageal variceal pressure assessed by endoscopic fine needle puncture under basal condition, Valsalva's manoeuvre and after glycyltrinitrate. *Gut* 1985; **26**: 525–530.

38 Bosch J, Bordas H, Rigau J *et al.* Non invasive measurement of the pressure of esophageal varices using an endoscopic gauge: comparison with measurement by variceal puncture in patients undergoing endoscopic sclerotherapy. *Hepatology* 1986; **6**: 667–672.

39 Kleber G, Sauerbruch T, Fischer G, Paumgartner G. Pressure of intraesophageal varices assessed by fine needle puncture: its relation to endoscopic signs and severity of liver disease in patients with cirrhosis. *Gut* 1989; **30**: 228–232.

40 Ohta M, Hashizume M, Higashi H *et al.* Portal and gastric mucosal hemodynamics in cirrhotic patients with portal-hypertensive gastropathy. *Hepatology* 1994; **20**: 1432–1436.

41 Taranto D, Suozzo R, Romano M *et al.* Gastric endoscopic features in patients with liver cirrhosis: correlation with esophageal varices, intravariceal pressure and liver dysfunction. *Digestion* 1994; **55**: 115–120.

42 El Gendi MA, Azzam ZA, Karara K *et al.* Effect of gastro-esophageal decongestion on variceal pressure in patients with schistosomal hepatic fibrosis. *Int Surg* 1994; **79**: 68–71.

43 Nevens F, Sprengers D, Fevery J. The effect of different doses of a bolus injection of somatostatin combined with a slow infusion on transmural esophageal variceal pressure in patients with cirrhosis. *J Hepatol* 1994; **20**: 27–31.

44 Saraya A, Sarin SK. Effects of intravenous nitroglycerin and metoclopramide on intravariceal pressure: a double-blind, randomized study. *Am J Gastroenterol* 1993; **77**: 1850–1853.

45 Feu F, Bordas JM, Luca A *et al.* Reduction of variceal pressure by propranolol: comparison of the effects on portal pressure and azygos blood flow in patients with cirrhosis. *Hepatology* 1993; **18**: 1082–1089.

46 Cestari R, Braga M, Missale G, Ravelli P, Burroughs AK. Hemodynamic effect of triglycyl-lysine-vasopressin (glypressin) on intravascular esophageal variceal pressure in patients with cirrhosis. A randomized placebo controlled trial. *J Hepatol* 1990; **10**: 205–210.

47 Kleber G, Sauerbruch T, Fischer G, Geigenberger G, Paumgartner G. Reduction of transmural esophageal variceal pressure by metoclopramide. *J Hepatol* 1991; **12**: 362–366.

48 Calès P, Braillon A, Jiron MI *et al.* Superior portosystemic collateral circulation estimated by azygos blood flow in patients with cirrhosis: lack of correlation with esophageal varices and gastrointestinal bleeding: effect of propranolol. *J Hepatol* 1984; **1**: 37–46.

49 Lebrec D. Methods to evaluate portal hypertension. *Gastroenterol Clin N Am* 1992; **21**: 50–53.

50 Garcia-Tsao G, Groszmann R, Fisher R, Conn H, Atterbury C, Glickmann M. Portal pressure, presence of gastroesophageal varices and variceal bleeding. *Hepatology* 1985; **5**: 419–424.

51 Triger D, Smart H, Hosking S, Johnson A. Prophylactic sclerotherapy for esophageal varices: long-term results of a single-center trial. *Hepatology* 1991; **13**: 117–123.

52 Groszmann R, Bosch J, Grace N *et al.* Hemodynamic events in a prospective ran-

domized trial of propranolol versus placebo in the prevention of a first variceal hemorrhage. *Gastroenterology* 1990; **99**: 1401–7.

53 Vorobioff J, Picabea E, Gamen M *et al.* Propranolol compared with propranolol plus isosorbide dinitrate in portal-hypertensive patients: long-term hemodynamic and renal effects. *Hepatology* 1993; **18**: 477–484.

54 Garcia-Pagan JC, Feu F, Navasa M *et al.* Long-term hemodynamic effects of iso-sorbide-5-mononitrate in patients with cirrhosis and portal hypertension. *J Hepatol* 1990; **11**: 189–195.

55 Ready JB, Robertson AD, Goff JS, Rector WG Jr. Assessment of the risk of bleeding from esophageal varices by continuous monitoring of portal pressure. *Gastro-enterology* 1991; **100**: 1403–1410.

56 Garcia-Pagàn JC, Feu F, Castells A *et al.* Circadian variations of portal pressure and variceal hemorrhage in patients with cirrhosis. *Hepatology* 1994; **19**: 595–601.

57 Merkel C, Bolognesi M, Bellon S *et al.* Prognostic usefulness of hepatic vein cathe-terization in patients with cirrhosis and esophageal varices. *Gastroenterology* 1991; **102**: 973–979.

58 Shiomi S, Kuroki T, Ueda T *et al.* Measurement of portal systemic shunting by oral and per-rectal administration of (I123)iodoamphetamine and clinical use of results. *Am J Gastroenterol* 1994; **89**: 86–91.

59 D'Arienzo A, Celentano L, Cimino L *et al.* Per-rectal portal scintigraphy with tech-netium-99m pertechnetate for the early diagnosis of cirrhosis in patients with chronic hepatitis. *J Hepatol* 1992; **14**: 188–193.

60 Urbain D, Muls V, Makhoul E, Ham HR. Prognostic value of thallium-201 per rectum scintigraphy in alcoholic cirrhosis. *J Nucl Med* 1994; **35**: 832–834.

61 Dao T, Elfadel S, Bouvard G, Bouvard N *et al.* Assessment of portal contribution to liver perfusion by quantitative sequential scintigraphy and Doppler ultrasound in alcoholic liver cirrhosis. Diagnostic value in the detection of portal hypertension. *J Clin Gastroenterol* 1993; **16**: 160–167.

Baveno II Consensus Statements: Imaging Techniques and Haemodynamic Measurements in Portal Hypertension

Luigi Bolondi (Chairman), Angelo Gatta, Roberto Groszmann, Didier Lebrec, Fréderic Nevens, Carlo Sabbà and Tilman Sauerbruch

1   Presence of portal hypertension must be searched for in all cirrhotic patients.

2   The techniques to be used routinely for a first-level approach to the assessment of portal hypertension in patients with cirrhosis without previous bleeding are:

* Endoscopy and ultrasonography, preferably with Doppler.

3   Other techniques, such as measurement of variceal pressure by indirect methods, should be used only within research protocols.

4   There is no consensus on which combination of parameters has to be utilized for the assessment of the risk of bleeding.

Most of the experts rely only on endoscopic findings (mainly variceal size). Other optional parameters to be associated to the endoscopic findings are: Child score, HVPG, variceal pressure and Doppler US.

5   Non-treated patients at low or intermediate bleeding risk must be followed up by endoscopy at 12-month intervals. Other additional techniques such as Doppler US or variceal pressure are used by a few experts at the same time interval.

6   At present, the main indication for the use of angiography is the evaluation of patients, candidates for surgery or when Doppler US is unsatisfactory.

Magnetic resonance angiography has a potential in this field but is still employed only in research protocols.

There are no clinical indications for the use of per-rectal scintigraphy or laser Doppler.

7   The efficacy of new pharmacological treatments must be evaluated by measurement of portal pressure (HVPG). Doppler US and variceal pressure measurement are also used by some experts and their value is under investigation.

8   There is no technique which can predict rebleeding when performed in the first days after a bleeding episode.

Drug Therapy for Portal Hypertension: a 5-Year Review

Lisa Ferayorni, John Polio and Roberto J. Groszmann

INTRODUCTION

Drug therapy of portal hypertension is primarily the treatment and prevention of variceal haemorrhage. The aim of therapy is to reduce oesophageal varix wall tension which is accomplished pharmacologically by decreasing transmural variceal pressure by a reduction in portal and variceal pressure. This may be accomplished by decreasing portal venous and/or porto-collateral blood flow or by reducing intrahepatic or portocollateral resistance. While flow is secondary in importance to abnormal resistance in the maintenance of portal hypertension, the pharmacological agents currently available for the treatment of portal hypertension primarily act by modulation of the hyperdynamic splanchnic circulation. Vasoconstrictors decrease portal pressure by reducing splanchnic arterial flow. Vasodilators ideally will reduce intrahepatic and/or portocollateral resistance. A miscellaneous group of drugs directly influence flow and pressure within the oesophagogastric collaterals or decrease portal flow and therefore pressure secondary to alterations in blood volume. The last 5 years have clearly seen a general acceptance of drug therapy for portal hypertension. This is not a fad that will wane away with time, but is an important advance in the medical treatment of a syndrome with a mortality as high as an acute myocardial infarction.

VASOCONSTRICTORS

Vasopressin (VP) analogues

Triglycyl-lysine vasopressin (tGLVP; terlipressin or glypressin), a hormonogen of lysine-VP, is a synthetic VP analogue composed of three glycyl residues and lysine-VP. Following intravenous administration, the glycyl residues are cleaved from the hormonogen by endothelial peptidases allowing slow, prolonged release of lysine-VP [1]. It was postulated that the maintenance of low blood levels of the active agent would minimize systemic toxicity. Early studies in normal dogs and in stable cirrhotic patients demonstrated that the systemic and splanchnic haemodynamic effects of tGLVP are similar to those of VP [2,3]. However, while the haemodynamic effects of tGLVP and VP are comparable, the side effects observed with tGLVP in patients studies may be of lesser severity [4].

Meta-analysis has demonstrated that tGLVP is superior to placebo in controlling variceal bleeding and is the only agent that has been shown to improve survival in variceal bleeding [5–8]. Pooled estimates have failed to demonstrate a greater efficacy for tGLVP over VP or VP plus nitroglycerine (NTG) in controlling bleeding or in reducing mortality from bleeding varices [9]. Nevertheless, tGLVP was associated with significant lower complications when compared with VP with or without NTG. Moreover, tGLVP alone or in combination with NTG is equally as effective as balloon tamponade [10,11], somatostatin [12,13] or octreotide [14] in controlling variceal haemorrhage.

Experimental studies in portal hypertensive rats have demonstrated impaired systemic and splanchnic vasoconstriction in response to VP during haemorrhage [15,16]. The hyporesponsiveness to VP may be associated with activation of endogenous vasoconstrictors and could be overcome with higher doses of VP. This hyporesponsiveness may explain the variable clinical efficacy of VP. In patients with cirrhosis due to hepatitis B, those with active variceal haemorrhage demonstrated an impaired reduction in portal pressure in response to VP compared with those who were clinically stable [17]. This was not confirmed in another study of 11 patients with alcoholic cirrhosis and active variceal haemorrhage [18]. VP- and tGLVP-induced systemic vasoconstriction were preserved in a small group of patients with upper gastrointestinal (GI) haemorrhage from variceal and non-variceal sites [19].

VP and tGLVP have been used in combination with vasodilators in order to potentiate reduction in portal pressure while minimizing systemic haemodynamic toxicity. In portal hypertensive dogs and cirrhotic patients, the addition of NTG to VP enhances the reduction in portal pressure induced by VP due to a decrease in portal venous resistance and reverses the adverse effects of VP on systemic haemodynamics [20,21]. A similar effect on systemic haemodynamics was observed with the addition of NTG to tGLVP in stable patients with hepatitis B cirrhosis [22]. Clinical studies have demonstrated fewer side effects and improved efficacy with VP–NTG compared with VP alone [23–25]. Isoproterenol [26] and ketanserin [27] reverse the systemic haemodynamic effects of VP without potentiating its effect on portal pressure in patients with cirrhosis.

Somatostatin (ST)/octreotide (OT)

Somatostatin is a naturally occurring tetradecapeptide that has been isolated from the hypothalamus, pancreatic and enteric epithelial cells (D cells). Octreotide is a synthetic octapeptide that, by virtue of a shared four-amino acid segment, has similar pharmacological activity with greater potency and longer duration of action in comparison with the natural compound.

Somatostatin has been shown to decrease splanchnic blood flow in normal subjects [28,29]. Somatostatin-induced splanchnic vasoconstriction began within 30 seconds with a maximum response occurring 90 seconds after the initiation of the infusion. This was felt to be consistent with a direct action on vascular smooth muscle. However, ST and OT, in an *in vitro* perfused mesenteric artery preparation from normal and portal hypertensive rats, did not increase splanchnic vascular resistance [30]. These data indicate that ST and OT are not direct vasoconstrictors. In portal vein-ligated (PVL) rats, ST induced a reduction in portal pressure by producing splanchnic vasoconstriction. This effect, which was associated with a marked reduction in glucagon secretion, was abolished when glucagon was infused simultaneously with ST at a rate that maintained baseline circulating glucagon levels [31]. Thus, these agents may increase vascular tone by inhibiting secretion of gut-derived vasodilatory peptides, such as glucagon, vasoactive intestinal peptide, substance P and calcitonin gene-related peptide. The actions of these peptides are mediated by endothelial-dependent and -independent mechanisms [32].

Splanchnic haemodynamic studies of ST in stable cirrhotic patients have yielded conflicting results with a variable reduction in wedged hepatic venous pressure (WHVP) despite a reduction in total hepatic blood flow (HBF) [33,34]. Somatostatin has been shown consistently to reduce azygous blood flow (AzBF) [35,36] whereas it has been reported to both decrease [37,38] and increase intravariceal pressure [39]. Octreotide decreases superior mesenteric artery blood flow in normal and cirrhotic patients as assessed by indwelling Doppler catheters [40]. However, as observed with ST, OT has a variable effect on WHVP [34] and intravariceal pressure [41,42], while it consistently reduces AzBF [43–45]. These and other studies indicate that ST and OT may have a preferential effect on the portocollateral circulation. While OT may exhibit little effect on portal pressure in stable, fasting states, it has been shown to prevent the postprandial increase in portal pressure induced by a 40 g protein meal [46]. Moreover, it has been shown that OT prevents postprandial splanchnic hyperaemia [47] which may explain OT's effect on preventing an increase in portal pressure postprandially. Whether these haemodynamic effects impact on incidence of variceal bleeding remains to be seen.

Recently, it has been demonstrated that bolus injection of ST induced a significant, although short-lived, reduction in gastric blood flow (as assessed by laser Doppler flowmetry) in cirrhotic patients with portal hypertensive gastropathy [48]. Thus, ST or its longer-acting analogue OT, could be potentially useful in treatment of bleeding portal hypertensive gastropathy.

Somatostatin infusion in stable cirrhotics has a modest effect on the systemic circulation with transient elevation in mean arterial pressure (MAP), mild reduction in cardiac output (CO) and bradycardia. Octreotide causes a transient reduction in CO with bolus administration which is ameliorated when it is administered by constant infusion [34]. Somatostatin has been reported to adversely effect renal function in cirrhotics, although this was observed with volume loading which may induce alterations in endogenous vasodilators and vasoconstrictors [49,50]. In another study, without volume loading, OT had a beneficial effect on renal function [51]. Octreotide ameliorated the hyperdynamic circulation in association with enhanced sodium and water excretion in PVL rats [52].

A number of studies have assessed the use of ST or OT in comparison with placebo or other modalities for the control of variceal haemorrhage. Burroughs et al. [53] demonstrated that ST, when administered as a 250 μg bolus followed by a 5-day infusion of 250 μg/h, controlled and prevented early rebleeding from varices in 64% of patients compared with 41% of patients in a placebo group. Valenzuela et al. [54] were unable to demonstrate a therapeutic benefit for ST compared with placebo. However, the 83% response rate in the placebo group was greater than that observed in any other study of variceal haemorrhage, raising the question of selection bias. Meta-analyses of the randomized controlled trials of ST determined that control of variceal bleeding was significantly greater with ST compared with controls, although a significant difference in mortality was not observed [34,55].

Several trials have compared ST with VP for the treatment of variceal bleeding [56–60]. Pooled estimates have shown a reduction in failure to control bleeding but not in mortality with ST [9]. Of note, there were almost no complications associated with ST. When compared with tGLVP [12,13], balloon tamponade [61,62] or sclerotherapy [63,64], ST is equally effective in controlling bleeding and in affecting survival. Recently, three randomized controlled trials have shown that a continuous infusion of ST is as effective as emergency sclerotherapy in arresting variceal bleeding and preventing early (5 days) rebleeding [65–67]. Clinical efficacy and mortality observed with OT for variceal haemorrhage is comparable with that observed with VP or tGLVP with or without nitrates, sclerotherapy and balloon tamponade [34]. Excluding one study, the complications associated with ST and OT have been significantly less severe and less frequent than those other modalities [34].

Beta-adrenergic blockers

The introduction of beta-adrenergic blockers to the treatment of portal hypertension [68] has been one of the most significant steps in the area of drug treatment of portal hypertension. Non-selective beta-adrenergic blockers induce splanchnic arteriolar vasoconstriction with a resultant decrease in portal venous flow and portal pressure. The reduction in portal venous flow is a consequence of both $beta_1$- and $beta_2$-adrenergic blockade. In cirrhotic patients, propranolol induced a 34% reduction in AzBF, concomitant with a 15–20% reduction in portal pressure [69].

In a double-blind, placebo-controlled study, the acute administration of intravenous propranolol significantly reduced oesophageal variceal pressure as measured endoscopically with a pressure-sensitive gauge [70]. Propranolol has been shown to prevent the development of portosystemic shunting in chronic murine schistosomiasis in a rat model of cirrhosis [71,72]. The reduction in portocollateral vessel radius (with the associated influence on wall tension) and preferential effect on portocollateral blood flow may account for the ability of non-selective beta-blockers to reduce the risk of variceal haemorrhage despite the limited reduction in portal pressure. Meta-analyses have demonstrated that, compared with controls, non-selective beta-blockers significantly decrease the incidence of initial variceal haemorrhage, fatal haemorrhage and recurrent variceal haemorrhage in patients with cirrhosis [73–77]. Whether non-selective beta-blockers favourably influence long-term survival has been controversial; however, a recent meta-analysis by Bernard *et al.* [76] found that, in patients who had suffered a variceal haemorrhage, beta-blockers significantly improved the mean survival rate at 2 years from 67 to 74%.

Approximately 25–30% of cirrhotic patients will not respond to propranolol with a reduction in portal pressure, despite evidence of systemic beta-adrenergic blockade [78,79]. The explanation for this remains unclear; however, it may be due to an increase in portocollateral resistance [80] or to an impairment in alpha-mediated splanchnic vasoconstriction as demonstrated in aged PVL rats [80].

Beta-blockers vs. endoscopic sclerotherapy

A number of studies have compared beta-blockers with sclerotherapy in preventing recurrent variceal haemorrhage [81–87]. Despite a reduced rebleeding rate with sclerotherapy in some studies, meta-analysis did not show any significant difference in rebleeding or survival rate between beta-blockers and sclerotherapy [77]. Moreover, because the incidence and severity of complications are significantly greater with sclerotherapy than propranolol, sclerotherapy should not be considered superior to beta-blockers in prevention of recurrent bleeding.

Beta-blockers plus endoscopic sclerotherapy vs. endoscopic sclerotherapy alone

Meta-analysis of the clinical trials comparing combined therapy with sclerotherapy alone for prevention of recurrent variceal bleeding found no significant difference in risk of recurrent variceal bleeding, survival rate, time for eradication of varices or recurrence of varices after eradication [77].

Beta-blockers alone vs. beta-blockers plus endoscopic sclerotherapy

In two controlled studies, the combination of propranolol and sclerotherapy was superior to propranolol alone in preventing recurrent bleeding (2-year follow-up), although there was no difference in survival rate between the two treatment groups [88,89].

Beta-adrenergic blockers plus nitrates and other combinations

The addition of NTG to propranolol further decreases portal pressure without influencing the increase in portocollateral resistance induced by propranolol in PVL rats [90]. The addition of isosorbide-5-mononitrate (Is-5-Mn) or isosorbide dinitrate (ISDN) to propranolol enhances the portal pressure-lowering effect of propranolol in patients with cirrhosis and can reduce portal pressure in patients who were non-responders to propranolol alone [91–93]. A significant reduction in AzBF was also observed with combination therapy. Mean arterial pressure was significantly decreased with the addition of nitrates whereas this was not observed in patients treated with propranolol alone. The decrease in arterial pressure was associated with the development of ascites or need for increased doses of diuretics in 57% of patients receiving propranolol and isosorbide dinitrate [93]. However, a significant impairment in renal function was not observed with the administration of propranolol and isosorbide-5-mononitrate for 3 months to 30 patients following an acute variceal haemorrhage [94]. Nipradilol, a non-selective beta-adrenergic blocker with nitrate-like vasodilating activity, reduces portal pressure in cirrhotic patients to an extent comparable with propranolol [95]. However, at the doses used in this study, MAP was not lowered and, thus, nipradilol was not exerting a nitrovasodilatory effect. The addition of serotonin antagonists [96,97], alpha$_2$-adrenergic antagonists [98] and diuretics [99] to propranolol have been shown to potentiate the portal pressure-lowering effect of propranolol in animal models of portal hypertension and cirrhotic patients. All these combinations should be tested further. However, they do not seem to add major advantages over a non-selective beta-blocker/nitrate combination. One clinical trial suggests that the combination of nitrates and beta-blockers may be more effective than beta-blockers alone in preventing first variceal haemorrhage [100].

Other vasoconstrictors

Glibenclamide is a sulphonylurea which has been shown to increase vascular tone in portal, hepatic artery and systemic territories in PVL [101] and cirrhotic [102] rats. In both studies, this led to reduced portal pressure and hyperdynamic circulation. Direct blockade of vascular adenosine triphosphate (ATP)-sensitive K^+ channels, which causes depolarization of the smooth-muscle cell membrane and calcium entry into the cell, is the proposed mechanism underlying glibenclamide's vasoconstrictive effect [102,103]. We have recently found that the splanchnic vasodilating activity due to a hyperpolarizing endothelial vasodilator, although important in the mesenteric vasculature, is not abnormally increased in portal hypertensive rats [104].

Unfortunately, glibenclamide also causes significant vasoconstriction of the hepatic artery [101,102] which could adversely affect liver function, although this was not evaluated. Moreover, the renovascular response to glibenclamide (same dose) is unclear – vasoconstriction was seen in one study [101] and no response in the other [101] – a discrepancy which was not explained.

VASODILATORS

Organic nitrates

Administration of short-acting (NTG) or long-acting (ISDN, Is-5-Mn) organic nitrates produces vasodilatation of vascular smooth muscle by forming nitric oxide and 5-nitrosothiol intracellularly, which stimulates guanylate cyclase to produce cyclic guanosine 3′,5′-monophosphate (cGMP). This inhibits intracellular calcium release from the sarcoplasmic reticulum, which reduces the cell's permeability to extracellular calcium, and hence, lowers the intracellular calcium concentration [105]. Organic nitrates have predominantly venodilatory effects with lesser effects on the arterial circulation [106]. Isosorbide-5-mononitrate, the vasoactive metabolite of ISDN, has minimal first-pass metabolism [107], whereas ISDN has a high first-pass effect [108], which makes the mononitrate the long-acting nitrate of choice in patients with hepatic insufficiency and portosystemic shunting.

Nitrates were introduced into the treatment of portal hypertension by using them in a combination with VP [20]. Since the initial report, several studies have demonstrated that the addition of NTG to VP enhances the reduction in portal pressure while counteracting the adverse systemic haemodynamic effects of VP [21–25,109]. Meta-analysis of three clinical trials has demonstrated that the combination of VP plus NTG is superior to VP alone in controlling variceal bleeding [9]. Soon after the introduction of the combination VP–NTG, it was recognized that NTG has portal hypotensive effects of its own.

The mechanisms by which organic nitrates reduce portal pressure have emerged primarily from studies in portal hypertensive animals. In portal hypertensive rats, NTG infusion significantly reduced portal pressure by reducing portal venous inflow [110,111]. This effect is the result of a baroreceptor-mediated splanchnic vasoconstriction induced by venous pooling and reduced arterial pressure. The reduction in portal pressure was enhanced when NTG and propranolol were administered together [111]. It has been demonstrated that the splanchnic effects of nitrates are dose-dependent [112]. Studies in isolated perfused cirrhotic rat livers have demonstrated that nitrates reduce intrahepatic vascular resistance [113,114].

Similar mechanisms may account for the portal hypotensive effect of nitrates observed in cirrhotic patients. Several studies have shown that both short- and long-term administration of nitrates can reduce the HVPG and/or portal pressure in patients with cirrhosis [115–127]. Although changes in MAP appear to correlate poorly with reduction in HVPG [119], Hayes *et al.* [121] found a significant correlation between the reduction in portal pressure gradient, the fall in cardiac index and the increase in systemic vascular resistance (at low doses). The effect of organic nitrates on the collateral circulation in cirrhotic patients has been variable and dose-dependent. An increase, a decrease or no change in AzBF have been observed after nitrate administration [117,123,124,126]. Taken together, haemodynamic studies performed in cirrhotic patients suggest that nitrates may decrease portal pressure by: (i) inducing a baroreflex-mediated splanchnic arterial vasoconstriction (paradoxical vasoconstriction) with a consequent reduction in portal venous flow; (ii) decreasing collateral resistance; (iii) reducing intrahepatic resistance; or most likely (iv) a variable combination of these mechanisms.

The variability in response to organic nitrates among patients with cirrhosis may be the result of different doses, variability in hepatic extraction, severity of liver disease or development of tolerance. Pharmacological tolerance to organic nitrates after chronic administration is well documented in patients with coronary artery disease [105]. Whether tolerance to nitrovasodilators also occurs in portal hypertensive cirrhotic patients is unclear.

The development of nitrate tolerance has been associated with a reduction of sulphhydryl groups in vascular smooth-muscle cells [105]. Blei and Gottstein [112] demonstrated an increased vascular responsiveness to organic nitrates in portal hypertensive rats given *n*-acetylcysteine (a sulphhydryl group donor). Whether a deficiency of sulphhydryl groups is responsible for 'non-responders' to organic nitrates in patients with cirrhosis is unknown. Several studies have demonstrated a sustained reduction in HVPG in patients with cirrhosis after chronic nitrate therapy [116,124,128,129], which argues against the development of full tolerance. However, tolerance may explain why Vorobioff *et al.* [129] found that three out of 10 cirrhotic patients had no reduction in HVPG after chronic ISDN administration. Furthermore, Garcia-Pagan *et al.* [124] demonstrated that in patients with cirrhosis, chronic oral administration of Is-5-Mn caused a modest but significant decrease in HVPG which was associated with the development of partial pharmacological tolerance (as shown by blunted haemodynamic response to intravenous NTG after chronic Is-5-Mn therapy). Grose *et al.* [126], on the other hand, found that 1-month administration of Is-5-Mn uniformly reduced AzBF but did not induce a sustained reduction in HVPG. Moreover, tolerance to nitrates was not observed in this study.

In a prospective randomized controlled trial, Angelico *et al.* [92] compared Is-5-Mn with propranolol in preventing first variceal haemorrhage in patients with cirrhosis and oesophageal varices documented by endoscopy. Isosorbide-5-mononitrate (20 mg per os, tid) was as safe and effective as propranolol (20–120 mg/day per os) in prophylaxis of first variceal bleeding. Patients without ascites at entry did not develop ascites during follow-up, nor did the requirement for diuretics change in patients with ascites. Of note, at the doses given in this study, long-term Is-5-Mn therapy had no adverse effects on liver or renal function, despite concerns raised by others [130]. Because diuretics were not discontinued in patients with ascites and this was not taken into account in the analysis of the data, the results of this study are difficult to interpret, particularly in light of several studies which have shown that diuretics can independently lower HVPG and portal pressure [131–134]. Also, the median dose of propranolol used in this study was lower than that used in previous studies. Furthermore, all patients simultaneously received ranitidine, a drug that may affect the metabolism of other drugs. Recently, Bertoni *et al.* [135] demonstrated that Is-5-Mn (50 mg/day per os) was more effective than placebo in reducing the rebleeding rate and the number of rebleeding episodes before variceal eradication with sclerotherapy in cirrhotic patients presenting with their first bleed from oesophageal varices.

Thus, the use of NTG to counteract the adverse haemodynamic effects of vasopressin in the treatment of acute variceal haemorrhage is recommended.

However, the role of chronic oral nitrates alone or in combination with other agents in the pharmacological management of portal hypertension still requires further investigation. In a recently reported prospective randomized trial, Villanueva et al. [136] demonstrated that combined administration of nadolol plus Is-5-Mn was more effective in preventing variceal rebleeding and was associated with fewer complications when compared with endoscopic sclerotherapy. Further controlled clinical trials are needed to confirm the efficacy of nitrates in preventing variceal haemorrhage and to elucidate their long-term effects on hepatic and renal function.

Other nitrovasodilators

Molsidomine is an antianginal drug with a predominant vasodilator effect on the venous system [137]. It is a pro-drug which is metabolized in the liver to its active form SIN-1 (linsidomine) and is transformed to SIN-1A in the blood, which in turn induces relaxation of vascular smooth muscle via stimulation of guanylate cyclase and cGMP formation [138]. The mechanism by which molsidomine reduces portal pressure is believed to be similar to other nitrovasodilators except, unlike organic nitrates, molsidomine does not induce tolerance and has minimal effects on the arterial pressure [138–141]. Molsidomine is believed to reduce portal pressure primarily by causing venodilatation which leads to a decrease in CO and MAP with resultant reflex splanchnic arterial vasoconstriction; and ultimately, a decrease in the portal venous inflow. No change in systemic vascular resistance is seen, as molsidomine has minimal effect on arteriolar smooth muscle [137]. Its haemodynamic effects are long-lasting and may be detectable for up to 6–8 hours after an oral dose [139].

Vinel et al. [137] studied the effect of a 4 mg oral dose of molsidomine in patients with alcoholic cirrhosis and portal hypertension. The HVPG was reduced by approximately 15%, mainly through a decrease of the WHVP. Mean arterial pressure, CO and HBF were also significantly decreased; however, hepatic clearance of indocyanine green did not change. In three out of 13 patients, molsidomine had no effect on the HVPG. Likewise, Ruiz del Arbol et al. [142] showed that oral administration of 2 and 4 mg of molsidomine to cirrhotic portal hypertensive patients caused an 11% and 10% reduction in the HVPG, respectively. Hepatic blood flow and, to a lesser extent, MAP and CO were decreased; however, there was no significant change in systemic vascular resistance. Using pulsed Doppler flow-metry, Monnin et al. [143] evaluated the effect of molsidomine and molsidomine plus propranolol in patients with cirrhosis and portal hypertension. Molsidomine significantly decreased portal blood flow velocity without decreasing systolic arterial pressure. A significant decrease in portal blood flow velocity was also observed after the addition of molsidomine to propranolol.

Desmorat *et al.* [144] found that there was a significant reduction in the portal venous pressure and MAP in linsidomine (active metabolite of molsidomine)-treated cirrhotic rats which was attributed to a drop in portocollateral and intrahepatic vascular resistances rather than to a reduction in total liver blood flow. The conclusions of this study must be interpreted with caution because, although there was a trend toward greater collateral blood flow and diminished portohepatic resistances in the linsidomine-treated rats, the differences did not reach statistical significance.

Chronic oral administration of molsidomine decreased sinusoidal pressure and variceal pressure in 85% of a small cohort of patients [145]. Although molsidomine has been shown to reduce the HVPG in patients with cirrhosis, there is a 13–28% 'non-responder' rate. Adverse side effects of molsidomine may include headache, facial flushing, orthostatic hypotension, GI distress and anorexia. Moreover, it is contraindicated in patients with glaucoma [139]. The clinical efficacy of this interesting compound remains to be demonstrated in controlled clinical trials.

Clonidine

Clonidine is an alpha$_2$-adrenergic agonist which inhibits central vasomotor centres, thereby decreasing sympathetic outflow from the central nervous system (CNS). This leads to reduced plasma catecholamine levels, plasma renin activity and peripheral vascular resistance [146]. Clonidine-induced inhibition of sympathetic outflow has been associated with a decrease in portal pressure and correction of the hyperdynamic circulation in both portal hypertensive animals [147] and in patients with cirrhosis [148–151].

In patients with alcoholic cirrhosis, acute administration of intravenous clonidine caused a significant decrease in both the HVPG and portal pressure without affecting HBF [148–151]. Additionally, Moreau *et al.* [149] demonstrated a 27% reduction in AzBF following clonidine administration, which could have an important effect in decreasing the risk of variceal bleeding. Because HBF was not reduced by clonidine, despite reduced CO and blood pressure (BP), Willet *et al.* [148] and Esler *et al.* [151] have suggested that the fall in portal pressure resulted from decreased postsinusoidal hepatic outflow resistance. Alternatively, clonidine-induced reduction in portal pressure could be by a passive mechanism resulting from reduced CO and MAP or by reflex splanchnic vasoconstriction secondary to decreased arterial pressure, both of which would reduce portal venous inflow [149]. In rats with sinusoidal portal hypertension due to bile duct ligation-induced cirrhosis, the acute administration of intravenous clonidine reduced portal pressure by decreasing portal venous inflow (resulting from splanchnic arteriolar vasoconstriction) [147]. In contrast to clinical studies in cirrhotic patients, in this animal model clonidine did not reduce CO or arterial pressure. In an isolated perfused liver preparation from cirrhotic rats, however, clonidine had no effect on intrahepatic vascular resistance [114].

In patients with alcoholic cirrhosis, chronic oral clonidine (0.30–0.45 mg/day to maintain systolic blood pressure (SBP) $\geqslant$ 100 mmHg) caused a significant reduction in the HVPG which was due entirely to a rise in free hepatic venous pressure (FHVP) [152]. Despite causing an equally significant decrease in the CO, arterial pressure and heart rate (HR), HBF, renal function and metabolic liver function were not adversely affected. In another study of eight patients with cirrhosis and ascites, chronic clonidine (150 μg/day for 1 week) decreased the HVPG by 10% which was due to a decrease in WHVP; however, the arterial pressure and CO were unchanged [153].

Thus, the mechanism by which clonidine lowers portal pressure and the potential problems it may cause from chronic reduction in arterial pressure need to be defined by further investigation before the drug can be recommended in the treatment of portal hypertension.

Serotonin blockers

It has been suggested that serotoninergic mechanisms may contribute to the maintenance of portal hypertension [154,155]. Serotonin is a potent venoconstrictor which has been shown to increase portal perfusion pressure and intrahepatic vascular resistance in isolated perfused liver of normal rats [156] and to increase portal resistance in normal dogs [157]. Furthermore, Cummings et al. [154,155] found that isolated superior mesenteric veins from portal hypertensive rats were hypersensitive to serotonin. Administration of ketanserin (a serotonin-receptor blocker) significantly reduced portal pressure in portal hypertensive rats. This decrease in portal pressure was due to a decrease in portal venous inflow, which resulted from venous pooling in the portal system and reduced CO [155]. The results of these studies suggested that ketanserin's portal pressure-lowering effect was primarily through serotonin blockade, although its alpha$_1$-adrenergic receptor antagonism and arterial hypotensive effect probably played a lesser role [155].

Two clinical studies have demonstrated that ketanserin significantly lowers portal pressure in patients with alcoholic cirrhosis and portal hypertension [158,159]. Unfortunately, this beneficial effect on portal pressure was accompanied by significant arterial hypotension after intravenous administration (10 mg) [158] and, with chronic oral administration (40–80 mg), reversible hepatic encephalopathy [159].

Two clinical studies examined combination therapy with ketanserin.

Hadengue *et al.* [160] investigated the acute haemodynamic effects of ketanserin with verapamil or propranolol in patients with alcoholic cirrhosis. To avoid arterial hypotension, a reduced dose of ketanserin (5 mg IV) was used. While ketanserin plus verapamil offered no beneficial effect over ketanserin alone in lowering portal pressure, ketanserin plus propranolol enhanced reductions in the WHVP, HVPG and AzBF and converted 'non-responders' to propranolol into 'responders'. Furthermore, neither ketanserin alone nor in combination with verapamil or propranolol caused arterial hypotension at the small dose used in this study. Lee *et al.* [161] evaluated the acute haemodynamic effects of intravenous VP (0.66 units/min) plus high-dose ketanserin (10 mg IV) in patients with compensated hepatitis B-related cirrhosis. Although ketanserin improved the adverse systemic haemodynamic effects of VP, it did not further reduce the portal pressure and induced a significant decrease in arterial pressure.

Ritanserin, a 5-hydroxytryptamine (5-HT$_2$) receptor blocker, has a higher binding affinity than ketanserin and no alpha$_1$-adrenoreceptor blocking effects [162]. Consequently, ritanserin does not cause arterial hypotension [163]. In several animal models of portal hypertension, ritanserin has been shown to decrease portal pressure without changing portal venous inflow. This suggests that its effect on portal pressure is mediated by a reduction in intrahepatic and/or portocollateral resistance [164–167]. Furthermore, in all of these studies, ritanserin lowered portal pressure without causing systemic hypotension. Similar results have been seen in a small group of patients with well-compensated cirrhosis wherein low-dose ritanserin (0.08 mg/kg/day for 7 days) significantly lowered portal pressure without causing arterial hypotension or hepatic encephalopathy [168]. A more recent study from this same group of investigators demonstrated that in cirrhotic rats, the portal pressure-lowering effect of ritanserin could be potentiated by the reduction of portal venous inflow induced by propranolol without affecting arterial pressure [169]. Further human investigations with ritanserin alone or in combination with another class of portal hypotensive agent are needed before determining whether selective serotonin blockers have any role in the treatment of portal hypertension.

Prasozin

In patients with advanced cirrhosis, chronic oral prazosin (an alpha-adrenoreceptor blocker) caused a significant reduction in the HVPG without significant effect on cardiac index, MAP or systemic vascular resistance [170]. Moreover, chronic prazosin was well tolerated in these patients, in that none of them developed renal impairment, sodium and water retention or hepatic encephalopathy. In portal hypertensive rats, acute administration of prazosin (5 μg/kg intraportal injection) had only a minimal effect on portal haemodynamics despite causing a 14% decrease in BP [155]. More recently, Albillos et al. [171] demonstrated that in patients with cirrhosis and portal hypertension, short-term oral prazosin significantly lowered the HVPG, whereas chronic prazosin did not further reduce portal pressure but worsened peripheral arterial vasodilatation and fluid retention. Tolerance was also seen after chronic prazosin therapy as it was necessary to double the dose to maintain a similar reduction in portal pressure. Because HBF was increased (statistically significant only for chronic therapy), these investigators concluded the prazosin lowered portal pressure by reducing the hepatic vascular resistance. By contrast, in isolated perfused cirrhotic rat livers, Marteau et al. [114] found that prazosin did not decrease intrahepatic vascular resistance. The mechanisms by which acute administration of prazosin lowers portal pressure is unclear. Reflex splanchnic vasoconstriction in response to arterial hypotension may contribute to a reduction in splanchnic arteriolar flow and hence portal pressure.

Calcium channel blockers

In perfused liver preparations from cirrhotic rats, high-dose verapamil decreased hepatic vascular resistance and portal perfusion pressure, with improvement in hepatic microvascular exchange and liver function [172, 173]. These authors speculate that verapamil's ability to decrease hepatic vascular resistance could be due to an effect on endothelial cells which ultimately regulate sinusoidal pressure. However, Marteau et al. [114], using a similar in vitro preparation, were unable to demonstrate a reduction in hepatic vascular resistance in response to verapamil, nifedipine or diltiazem.

In cirrhotic patients, acute intravenous administration of verapamil caused a small but significant fall in the HVPG without significant systemic haemodynamic effects [116]. In another study [174], acute intravenous verapamil caused a 14% decrease in HVPG (secondary to a decrease in WHVP) in patients with HBsAg-positive cirrhosis which was sustained in chronic oral therapy. Arterial pressure decreased but CO and HR were not affected. Direct measurements of portal venous pressure and HBF were not assessed. Unfortunately, it was difficult to interpret these results because in patients with non-alcoholic cirrhosis, WHVP can significantly underestimate portal pressure [175,176]. However, recent reports have found that WHVP measurement may not underestimate the severity of portal hypertension in all forms of non-alcoholic cirrhosis [177,178]. In 21 patients with hepatitis B-related cirrhosis, Lin et al. [177] found an excellent correlation between portal venous pressure and WHVP. After analysing the data of 40 patients with non-alcoholic cirrhosis from four of their previously published studies, Iwao *et al.* [178] found that the WHVP accurately reflected portal venous pressure during vasoactive drug administration in these patients.

Multiple studies in patients with alcoholic cirrhosis have failed to document any reduction in portal pressure or improvement in liver function with calcium channel blockers [160,179–181]. Indeed, nifedipine has been shown to increase the HVPG in patients with cirrhosis [182]. Iwao *et al.* [183] demonstrated that continuous infusion of nicardipine, a new calcium channel blocker, increased hepatic blood flow and improved hepatic function, but had no beneficial effect on portal pressure in cirrhotic patients. In another study by the same group, the addition of nicardipine to VP improved the adverse haemodynamic effects of VP but caused no further reduction in portal pressure in a group of 18 patients with cirrhosis [184]. Garcia-Pagan *et al.* [185] demonstrated that the acute oral administration of nicardipine increased HBF and hepatic clearance of indocyanine green in patients with cirrhosis without lowering the HVPG. Moreover, nicardipine significantly increased AzBF which could be detrimental in patients with oesophageal varices and portosystemic encephalopathy. Therefore, given the evidence thus far, it is not clear that calcium channel blockers have any role in the pharmacological treatment of portal hypertension.

DRUGS WHICH INCREASE LOWER OESOPHAGEAL SPHINCTER PRESSURE

Miskowiak [186] first suggested that the administration of drugs that increase the lower oesophageal sphincter pressure might reduce the inflow of blood into oesophageal varices. Portographic studies in patients with cirrhosis and portal hypertension have shown that pentagastrin, metoclopramide and domperidone – all drugs which increase lower oesophageal sphincter tone – can significantly reduce blood flow to oesophageal varices [187–189]. In support of these studies, Mastai *et al.* [190] demonstrated that metoclopramide and domperidone, but not placebo, reduced the AzBF in patients with cirrhosis without affecting portal pressure, HBF or systemic haemodynamics. These authors concluded that by increasing the lower oesophageal sphincter pressure, these drugs could reduce the inflow of blood into oesophageal varices. By contrast, in two much smaller studies in cirrhotic patients, the same dose of domperidone, although effective in raising the lower oesophageal sphincter tone, did not significantly affect AzBF [191] nor decrease blood flow into oesophageal varices [192]. These discrepant results may be explained by the different timing that AzBF was measured after administration of drug. The effects of domperidone were only measured at 15 minutes in the study by Braillon *et al.* [191], whereas Mastai *et al.* [190]

demonstrated that the maximal effect of domperidone and metoclopramide on AzBF was seen at 40 minutes.

Controversy also exists as to whether metoclopramide significantly reduces variceal pressure. In patients with cirrhosis and portal hypertension [193–195], intravenous metoclopramide (10–20 mg) caused significant reductions in oesophageal variceal pressure as measured endoscopically by direct puncture of the varices, although others [196] were not able to confirm these results. Moreover, metoclopramide at a dose of 20 mg IV [197] but not 10 mg IV [193] caused a small but significant reduction in portal blood flow as measured by pulsed Doppler ultrasonography. In two small clinical studies, intravenous administration of metoclopramide (20 mg) was effective in stopping active oesophageal variceal bleeding by constricting the lower oesophageal sphincter [198,199]. However, in a prospective, randomized trial, domperidone and metoclopramide were not more effective than placebo in preventing early variceal rebleeding in patients with cirrhosis [200]. Most interesting, however, is the recent study by Ohta *et al.* [201] which demonstrated that repeat intraperitoneal injection of high-dose metoclopramide (15 mg/kg daily), for 14 days, to portal hypertensive rats prevented the development of oesophageal varices by causing constriction of the lower oesophageal sphincter. These authors point out that such a high dose of metoclopramide could be hazardous to cirrhotic patients because of its potential to worsen sodium retention. Indeed, in agreement with previous findings in normal subjects [202,203], D'Arienzo *et al.* [204] demonstrated in a group of cirrhotic patients with ascites that metoclopramide, but not domperidone, significantly increased plasma aldosterone levels and impaired the natriuretic response to spironolactone. Consequently, metoclopramide should be used with caution in patients with ascites [205]. Because domperidone may be more effective than metoclopramide in lowering variceal blood flow [190] and does not impair diuresis in patients with cirrhosis [204], future clinical trials should evaluate the efficacy of domperidone rather than metoclopramide in preventing oesophageal varices or variceal haemorrhage. The effect of cisapride (a longer-acting drug which increases lower oesophageal sphincter tone) on oesophageal variceal haemodynamics has not been reported to date.

DIURETICS

Sodium retention and plasma volume expansion, a common finding in patients with chronic liver diseases, contributes to the severity of portal hypertension [206–208]. Plasma volume depletion induced by sodium restriction and/or diuretics leads to decreased portal pressure in patients with cirrhosis [209–212] and in portal hypertensive animals [213] and improves the hyperdynamic circulatory state [213,214]. Several clinical studies have demonstrated that both acute and chronic administration of diuretics, including spironolactone and furosemide, significantly reduce plasma volume, portal pressure and/or the HVPG [209–212]. From these studies, it appears that the mechanism by which diuretics reduce the HVPG and portal pressure is by reducing circulating plasma volume which decreases CO which, in turn, induces a baroreceptor-mediated reflex splanchnic vasoconstriction. The resultant decrease in splanchnic arterial blood flow results in a decrease in portal pressure and AzBF.

Different diuretics have had variable effects on portal pressure and AzBF. Acute administration of furosemide (0.75 mg/kg IV) significantly reduced CO, AzBF and the HVPG in cirrhotic patients not receiving beta-blockers [211]. Similar effects on AzBF and HVPG were not observed in patients who were taking beta-blockers despite a significant decrease in blood volume and CO [215]. Although acute administration of furosemide to cirrhotic patients on chronic beta-blocker therapy does not appear to further decrease portal pressure [215], the potential long-term effects of this combination on portal hypertension remain to be seen.

Chronic administration of spironolactone but not furosemide significantly reduced the WHVP [212,216], the HVPG [212,216,217] and AzBF [217] in cirrhotic patients without ascites without adversely affecting HBF [217]. In these studies the reduction in portal pressure appeared to be secondary to plasma volume contraction. The acute addition of intravenous propranolol to the chronic spironolactone therapy further reduced the HVPG [217]. Taken together, these studies suggest that long-term therapy with spironolactone alone or in combination with propranolol may be useful in the treatment of portal hypertension in cirrhotic patients without ascites.

Recently, Garcia-Pagan *et al.* [214] examined the haemodynamic effects of spironolactone (100 mg daily) and low-sodium diet (50 mEq daily) or low-sodium diet alone in patients with compensated cirrhosis and portal hypertension. Spironolactone plus a low-sodium diet but not salt restriction alone significantly reduced plasma volume, CO, portal pressure and AzBF without adversely affecting HBF or renal function. By contrast, in an animal model of portal hypertension, sodium restriction alone caused a significant reduction in plasma volume and ameliorated the hyperdynamic circulation [213].

The main limitation to the use of diuretics in the pharmacological management of portal hypertension appears to be their potential adverse effects on renal function.

FUTURE STUDIES

There are now a number of drug combinations that seem to be very effective in reducing portal pressure. Whether these more effective therapies will be reflected in an increased efficacy in preventing variceal bleeding and rebleeding and an increasing survival remains to be proved by future clinical trials.

REFERENCES

1 Cort JH, Albrecht I, Novakova J, Mulder JL, Jost K. Regional and systemic haemo-dynamic effects of some vasopressins: structural features of the hormone which prolongs activity. *Eur J Clin Invest* 1975; **5**: 165–175.
2 Blei AT, Groszmann RJ, Gusberg RJ, Conn HO. Comparison of vasopressin and triglycyl-lysine vasopressin on splanchnic and systemic hemodynamics in dogs. *Dig Dis Sci* 1980; **25**: 688–694.
3 Rabol A, Juhl E, Schmidt A, Winkler K. The effect of vasopressin and triglycyl-vasopressin (glypressin) on the splanchnic circulation in cirrhotic patients with portal hypertension. *Digestion* 1976; **14**: 285–289.
4 D'Amico G, Traina M, Vizzini G *et al.* Terlipressin or vasopressin plus transdermal nitroglycerin in the treatment strategy for digestive bleeding in cirrhosis. A rando-mized clinical trial. *J Hepatol* 1994; **20**: 206–212.
5 Walker S, Stiehl A, Raedsch R, Kommerell B. Terlipressin in bleeding esophageal varices: a placebo controlled, double-blind study. *Hepatology* 1986; **6**: 112–115.
6 Freeman JG, Cobden MD, Record CO. Placebo-controlled trial of terlipressin (Glypressin) in the management of acute variceal bleeding. *J Clin Gastroenterol* 1989; **11**: 58–60.
7 Soederlund C, Magnusson I, Torngren S, Lundell L. Terlipressin (triglycyl-lysine vasopressin) controls acute bleeding oesophageal varices. A double-blind, rando-mized, placebo-controlled trial. *Scand J Gastroenterol* 1990; **25**: 622–630.
8 Freeman JG, Cobden I, Lishman AH, Record CO. Controlled trial of terlipressin ('glypressin') versus vasopressin in the early treatment of esophageal varices. *Lancet* 1982; **ii**: 66–69.
9 Bosch J, D'Amico G, Luca A, Garcia-Pagan JC, Feu F, Escorsell A. Drug therapy for variceal hemorrhage. In: Bosch J, Groszmann RJ (eds), *Portal Hypertension: Patho-physiology and Treatment*. Oxford: Blackwell Scientific Publications, 1994: 108–123.
10 Colin R, Giuli N, Czernichow P, Ducrotte P, Lerebours E. Prospective comparison of glypressin, tamponade, and their association in the treatment of bleeding esophageal varices. In: Lebrec D, Blei AT (eds), *Vasopressin Analogs and Portal Hypertension*. Paris: John Libbey Eurotext, 1987: 149–153.
11 Fort E, Sautereau D, Silvain C, Ingrand P, Pillegand B, Beauchant M. A randomized trial of terlipressin plus nitroglycerin vs balloon tamponade in the control of acute variceal hemorrhage. *Hepatology* 1990; **11**: 678–681.
12 Walker S, Kreichgauer HP, Bode JC. Terlipressin vs somatostatin in bleeding eso-phageal varices: a controlled double blind study. *Hepatology* 1992; **15**: 1023–1030.
13 Variceal Bleeding Study Group. Double blind comparison of somatostatin infusion vs glypressin injection in the treatment of acute variceal haemorrhage in patients with cirrhosis. *J Hepatol* 1993; **18** (Suppl. 1): 537A.

14 Silvain C, Carpentier S, Sautereau D *et al.* Terlipressin plus transdermal nitroglycerin vs. octreotide in the control of acute bleeding from esophageal varices: a multicenter randomized trial. *Hepatology* 1993; **18**: 61–65.

15 Kravetz D, Cummings SA, Groszmann RJ. Hyposensitivity to vasopressin in a hemorrhaged-transfused rat model of portal hypertension. *Gastroenterology* 1987; **93**: 170– 175.

16 Valla D, Girod C, Lee SS, Braillon A, Lebrec D. Lack of vasopressin action on splanchnic hemodynamics during bleeding: a study in conscious, portal hypertensive rats. *Hepatology* 1988; **8**: 10–15.

17 Tsai YT, Lee FY, Lin HC *et al.* Hyposensitivity to vasopressin in patients with hepatitis B-related cirrhosis during acute variceal hemorrhage. *Hepatology* 1991; **13**: 407–412.

18 Ready JB, Robertson AD, Rector WH. Effects of vasopressin on portal pressure during hemorrhage from esopageal varices. *Gastroenterology* 1991; **100**: 1411–1416.

19 Berling R, Aronsen KF, Rosberg B. Hemodynamic effects of triglycyl-lysine vasopressin and arginin vasopressin in patients with upper gastrointestinal bleeding. In: Lebrec D and Blei AT (eds), *Vasopressin Analogs and Portal Hypertension*. Paris: John Libbey Eurotex, 1987: 135–137.

20 Groszmann RJ, Kravetz, Bosch J *et al.* Nitroglycerin improves the hemodynamic response to vasopressin in portal hypertension. *Hepatology* 1982; **6**: 757–762.

21 Iwao T, Toyonaga A, Ikegami M *et al.* Portohepatic pressures, hepatic function, and blood gasses in the combination of nitroglycerin and vasopressin: search for additive effects in cirrhotic portal hypertension. *Am J Gastroenterol* 1992; **87**: 719–724.

22 Lin H-C, Tsai Y-T, Lee F-Y *et al.* Systemic and portal haemodynamic changes following triglycyllysine vasopressin plus nitroglycerin administration in patients with hepatitis B-related cirrhosis. *J Hepatol* 1990; **10**: 370–374.

23 Tsai YT, Lay CS, Lai KH *et al.* Controlled trial of vasopressin plus nitroglycerin vs vasopressin alone in the treatment of bleeding esophageal varices. *Hepatology* 1986; **6**: 406–409.

24 Gimson AES, Westaby D, Hegarty J, Alastair W, Williams R. A randomized trial of vasopressin plus nitroglycerin in the control of acute variceal hemorrhage. *Hepatology* 1986; **6**: 410–413.

25 Bosch J, Groszmann RJ, Garcia-Pagan JC *et al.* Association of transdermal nitroglycerin to vasopressin infusion in the treatment of variceal hemorrhage: a placebo-controlled trial. *Hepatology* 1989; **10**: 962–968.

26 Sirinek KR, Thomford NR. Isoproterenol in offsetting adverse effects of vasopressin in cirrhotic patients. *Am J Surg* 1975; **129**: 130–136.

27 Lee FY, Tsai YT, Lin HC *et al.* Hemodynamic effects of a combination of vasopressin and ketanserin in patients with hepatitis B-related cirrhosis. *J Hepatol* 1992; **15**: 54–58.

28 Wahren J, Felig P. Influence of somatostatin on carbohydrate disposal and absorption in diabetes mellitus. *Lancet* 1976; **2**: 1213–1216.

29 Sonneburg GE, Keller U, Perruchoud A *et al.* Effect of somatostatin on splanchnic hemodynamics in patients with cirrhosis of the liver and in normal subjects. *Gastroenterology* 1981; **80**: 526–532.

30 Sieber CC, Mosca PG, Groszmann RJ. Effect of somatostatin on mesenteric vascular resistance in normal and hypertensive rats. *Am J Physiol* 1992; **262**: 274–277.

31 Pizcueta MP, Garcia-Pagan JC, Fernandez M *et al.* Glucagon hinders the effects of

somatostatin on portal hypertension. A study in rats with partial portal vein ligation. *Gastroenterology* 1991; **101**: 1710–1715.

32 Rodriguez-Perez F, Groszmann RJ. Pharmacological treatment of portal hypertension. Groszmann RJ, Grace ND (eds), *Gastroenterology Clinics of North America* 1992, **21**(1): 15–40.

33 Polio J, Groszmann RJ. Pharmacological control of portal hypertension. In: Boyer J, Ockner R (eds), *Progress in Liver Diseases*. Philadelphia: WB Saunders Co, 1993: 231–249.

34 Burroughs AK. Octreoctide in variceal bleeding. *Gut* 1994; **38**: 523–527.

35 Bosch J, Kravetz D, Rodes J. Effects of somatostatin on hepatic and systemic hemodynamics in patients with cirrhosis of the liver: comparison with vasopressin. *Gastroenterology* 1981; **80**: 518–525.

36 Mastai R, Bosch J, Navasa M *et al.* Effect of continuous infusion and bolus injection of somatostatin on azygous blood flow and hepatic and systemic hemodynamics in patients with portal hypertension. Comparison with vasopressin (abstract). *J Hepatol* 1986; **3** (Suppl. 1): S53.

37 Clements D, Rhodes JM, Elias E. Effect of somatostatin on oesophageal variceal pressure assessed by direct measurement. *J Hepatol* 1986; **2**: 262–266.

38 Jenkins SA, Baxter JN, Corbett WA, Shields R. Effects of a somatostatin analogue SMS 201-995 on hepatic haemodynamics in the pig and on intravariceal pressure in man. *Br J Surg* 1985; **72**: 1009–1012.

39 Kleber G, Suerbruch T, Fischer G, Paumgarter G. Somatostatin does not reduce oesophageal variceal pressure in liver cirrhosis. *Gut* 1988; **29**: 153–156.

40 MacCormack PA, Seifalian AM, Stansby G *et al.* Superior mesenteric artery blood flow in man measured with intra-arterial Doppler catheters: effect of octreotide. *J Hepatol* 1993; **17**: 20–27.

41 Primignani M, Nolte A, Vazzoler MC *et al.* The effect of octreotide on intraoesophageal variceal pressure (IOVP) in liver cirrhosis is unpredictable (abstract). *Hepatology* 1990; **12**: A989.

42 Baxter JN, Jenkins SA, Shields R. SMS 210–995 and variceal hemorrhage. *Acta Endocrinol* 1987; S286: 37.

43 Navasa M, Bosch J, Chesta J *et al.* Haemodynamic effects of subcutaneous administration of SMS 201–995 a long acting somatostatin analogue in patients with cirrhosis and portal hypertension (abstract). *J Hepatol* 1988; **7** (Suppl. 1): S64.

44 Ericksson LS, Brundin T, Søderlund C, Wahren J. Haemodynamic effects of a long-acting somatostatin analogue in patients with liver cirrhosis. *Scand J Gastroenterol* 1987; **22**: 919–925.

45 MacCormick PA, Dick R, Siringo S *et al.* Octreotide reduces azygous blood flow in cirrhotic patients with portal hypertension. *Eur J Gastroenterol Hepatol* 1990; **2**: 489–492.

46 MacCormick PA, Biagini MR, Dick R *et al.* Octreotide inhibits the meal-induced increases in the portal venous pressure in cirrhotic patients with portal hypertension: a double blind, placebo controlled study. *Hepatology* 1992; **16**: 1180–1186.

47 Buonamico P, Sabbà C, Garcia-Tsao G *et al.* Octreotide blunts postprandial splanchnic hyperemia in cirrhotic patients: a double-blind randomized echo-Doppler study. *Hepatology* 1995; **21**: 134–139.

48 Panes J, Pique JM, Bordas JM *et al.* Effect of bolus injection and continuous infusion of somatostatin on gastric perfusion in cirrhotic patients with portal-hypertensive gastropathy. *Hepatology* 1994; **20** 336–341.

49 Gines A, Salmeron JM, Gines P *et al.* Effects of somatostatin on renal function in cirrhosis. *Gastroenterology* 1992; **103**: 1868–1874.

50 Dudley FJ. Somatostatin and portal hypertensive bleeding: a safe therapeutic alternative? *Gastroenterology* 1992; **103**: 1973–1977.

51 Mountokalakis T, Kallivretakis N, Mayopoulou-Symvoulidou D, Karvountzis G, Tolis G. Enhancement of renal function by a long-acting somatostatin analogue in patients with decompensated cirrhosis. *Nephrol Dial Transplant* 1988; **3**: 604–607.

52 Albillos A, Colombato LA, Lee FY *et al.* Octreotide ameliorates vasodilation and Na$^+$retention in portal hypertensive rats. *Gastroenterology* 1993; **104**: 575–579.

53 Burroughs AK, McCormick PA, Hughes MD *et al.* Randomized, double blind, placebo-controlled trial of somatostatin for variceal bleeding. *Gastroenterology* 1990; **99**: 1388–1395.

54 Valenzuela JE, Schubert T, Ronald Fogel M *et al.* A multicenter randomized, double-blind trial of somatostatin in the management of acute hemorrhage from esophageal varices. *Hepatology* 1989; **10**(6): 958–961.

55 Rojter S, Santarelli MT, Albornoz L, Mastai R. Somatostatin in acute variceal bleeding: a meta-analysis study. *J Hepatol* 1993; **19**: 189–190 (Letter).

56 Kravetz D, Bosch J, Teres J, Bruix J, Rimola AM, Rodes J. Comparison of intravenous somatostatin and vasopressin infusion in treatment of acute variceal hemorrhage. *Hepatology* 1984; **4**: 442–446.

57 Jenkins SA, Baxter JN, Corbett WA, Devitt P, Ware J, Shields R. A prospective randomized controlled clinical trial comparing somatostatin and vasopressin in controlling acute variceal haemorrhage. *Br Med J* 1985; **290**: 275–278.

58 Hsia HC, Lee FY, Tsai YT *et al.* Comparison of somatostatin and vasopressin in the control of acute esophageal variceal hemorrhage. A randomized, controlled study. *Chin J Gastroenterol* 1990; **7**: 71–78.

59 Saari A, Klvilaakso E, Inberg M *et al.* Comparison of somatostatin and vasopressin in bleeding esophageal varices. *Am J Gastroenterol* 1990; **85**: 804–807.

60 Rodriguez-Moreno F, Santolaria F, Glez-Reimers E *et al.* A randomized trial of somatostatin vs. vasopressin plus nitroglycerin in the treatment of acute variceal bleeding (abstract). *J Hepatol* 1991; **13**: S162.

61 Jaramillo JL, de la Mata M, Mino G, Costan G, Gomez-Camacho F. Somatostatin versus Sengstaken balloon tamponade for primary haemostasia of bleeding esophageal varices. *J Hepatol* 1991; **12**: 100–105.

62 Avgerinos A, Klonis C, Rekoumis G, Gouma P, Papedimitriou N. Controlled trial of somatostatin and balloon tamponade in bleeding esophageal varices. *J Hepatol* 1991; **13**: 78–83.

63 Di Febo G, Siringo S, Vacirca M *et al.* Somatostatin and urgent sclerotherapy in active esophageal variceal bleeding (abstract). *Gastroenterology* 1990; **98**: A583.

64 Planas R, Quer JQ, Boix J *et al.* Somatostatin and sclerotherapy in the treatment of acute variceal bleeding. A prospective randomized trial (abstract). *Gastroenterology* 1992; **102**: 279.

65 Shields R, Jenkins SA, Baxter JN *et al.* A prospective randomised controlled trial comparing the efficacy of somatostatin with injection sclerotherapy in the control of oesophageal varices. *J Hepatol* 1992; **16**: 128–137.

66 Variceal Bleeding Study Group. Randomized controlled trial of sclerotherapy versus somatostatin infusion in the prevention of early rebleeding following acute variceal hemorrhage in patients with cirrhosis. *Hepatology* 1993; **18**: 140A.

67 Planas R, Quer JC, Boix J *et al.* A prospective randomized trial comparing soma-

tostatin and sclerotherapy in the treatment of acute variceal bleeding. *Hepatology* 1994; **20**: 370–375.

68 Lebrec D, Nouel O, Corbic M, Benamou J-P. Propranolol – a medical treatment for portal hypertension. *Lancet* 1980; **ii**: 180–182.

69 Bosch J, Mastai R, Kravetz D *et al.* Effects of propranolol on azygous venous blood flow and hepatic and systemic hemodynamics in cirrhosis. *Hepatology* 1984; **4**: 1200–1205.

70 Feu F, Bordas JM, Garcia-Pagan JC, Bosch J, Rodes J. Double-blind investigation of the effects of propranolol and placebo on the pressure of esophageal varices in patients with portal hypertension. *Hepatology* 1991; **13**: 917–922.

71 Sarin SK, Groszmann RJ, Mosca PG *et al.* Propranolol ameliorates the development of portal-systemic shunting in a chronic murine schistosomiasis model of portal hypertension. *J Clin Invest* 1991; **87**: 1032–1036.

72 Colombato LA, Albillos A, Genecin P *et al.* Prevention of portal-systemic shunting in propranolol-treated and in sodium-restricted cirrhotic rats. *Gastroenterology* 1991; **100**: A730.

73 Hayes PC, Davis JM, Lewis JA, Bouchier IAD. Meta-analysis of value of propranolol in prevention of variceal hemorrhage. *Lancet* 1990; **335**: 153–156.

74 Pagliaro L, D'Amico G, Soerensen TIA *et al.* Prevention of first bleeding in cirrhosis. A meta-analysis of randomized trials of nonsurgical treatment. *Ann Intern Med* 1992; **117**: 59–70.

75 Poynard T, Cales P, Pasta L *et al.* Beta-adrenergic antagonist drugs in the prevention of gastrointestinal bleeding in patients with cirrhosis and esophageal varices. An analysis of data and prognostic factors in 589 patients from four randomized clinical trials. *N Engl J Med* 1991; **324**: 1532–1538.

76 Bernard B, Lebrec D, Mathurin P, Opolon P, Poynard T. Meta-analysis of beta-blockers in the prevention of recurrent variceal bleeding in patients with cirrhosis. *Hepatology* 1994; **20**: 106A.

77 Pagliaro L, Burroughs AK, Soerensen TIA *et al.* Therapeutic controversies and randomised controlled trials (R C Ts): prevention of bleeding and rebleeding in cirrhosis. *Gastroenterol Int* 1989; **2**: 71–84.

78 Garcia-Tsao G, Grace ND, Groszmann RJ *et al.* Short term effects of propranolol on portal venous pressure. *Hepatology* 1986; **6**: 101–106.

79 Lebrec D, Braillon A, Cales P *et al.* Influence of the stage of liver disease on systemic and splanchnic hemodynamics and on response to propranolol in patients with cirrhosis. *Hepatology* 1984; **4**: 1026A.

80 Polio J, Sieber CC, Lerner E *et al.* Cardiovascular hyporesponsiveness to norepinephrine, propranolol and nitroglycerin in portal hypertensive and aged rats. *Hepatology* 1993; **18**: 128–56.

81 Fleig WE, Stange EF, Hunecke R *et al.* Prevention of recurrent bleeding in cirrhotics with recent variceal hemorrhage: prospective, randomized comparison of propranolol and sclerotherapy. *Hepatology* 1987; **7**: 355–361.

82 Alexandrino PT, Alves MM, Pinto Carreia J. Propranolol or endoscopic sclerotherapy in the prevention of recurrence of variceal bleeding. A prospective, randomized controlled trial. *J Hepatol* 1988; **7**: 175–185.

83 Rossi VV, Cales P, Burtin P *et al.* Prevention of recurrent variceal bleeding in alcoholic cirrhotic patients: prospective controlled trial of propranolol and sclerotherapy. *J Hepatol* 1991; **12**: 283–289.

84 Qureshi H, Zuberi SJ, Alan E. Efficacy of oral propranolol and injection sclerotherapy

in the long-term management of variceal bleeding. *Digestion* 1990; **46**: 193–198.

85 Westaby D, Polson RJ, Gimson AES, Hayes PC, Hayllar K, Williams R. A controlled trial of oral propranolol compared with injection sclerotherapy for the long-term management of variceal bleeding. *Hepatology* 1990; **11**: 353–359.

86 Dasarathy S, Dwivedi M, Bhargava DK, Sundaram KR, Ramachandran K. A prospective randomized trial comparing repeated endoscopic sclerotherapy and propranolol in decompensated (Child class B and C) cirrhotic patients. *Hepatology* 1992; **16**: 89–94.

87 Teres J, Bosch J, Bordas JM *et al.* Propranolol versus sclerotherapy in preventing variceal rebleeding: a randomized controlled trial. *Gastroenterology* 1993; **105**: 1508–1514.

88 O'Connor KW, Lehman G, Yune H *et al.* Comparison of three nonsurgical treatments of bleeding esophageal varices. *Gastroenterology* 1989; **96**: 899–906.

89 Ink O, Martin T, Poynard T *et al.* Does elective sclerotherapy improve the efficacy of long-term propranolol for prevention of recurrent bleeding in patients with severe cirrhosis? A prospective multicenter, randomized trial. *Hepatology* 1992; **16**: 912–919.

90 Kroeger RJ, Groszmann RJ. The effect of the combination of nitroglycerin and propranolol on splanchnic and systemic hemodynamics in a portal hypertensive rat model. *Hepatology* 1985; **5**: 425–430.

91 Garcia-Pagan JC, Navasa M, Bosch J, Bru C, Pizcueta P, Rodes J. Enhancement of portal pressure reduction by association of isosorbide-5-mononitrate to propranolol administration in patients with cirrhosis. *Hepatology* 1990; **11**: 230–238.

92 Angelico M, Carli L, Piat C *et al.* Isosorbide-5-mononitrate versus propranolol in the prevention of first bleeding in cirrhosis. *Gastroenterology* 1993; **104**: 1460–1465.

93 Vorobioff J, Picabea E, Gamen M *et al.* Propranolol compared with propranolol plus isosorbide dinitrate in portal-hypertensive patients: long-term hemodynamic and renal effects. *Hepatology* 1993; **18**: 477–484.

94 Morillas RM, Planas R, Cabre E *et al.* Propranolol plus isosorbide-5-mononitrate for portal hypertension in cirrhosis: long-term hemodynamic and renal effects. *Hepatology* 1994; **20**: 1502–1508.

95 Aramaki T, Sekiyama T, Katsuta Y *et al.* Long-term haemodynamic effects of a 4-week regimen of nipradilol, a new β-blocker with nitrovasodilating properties, in patients with portal hypertension due to cirrhosis. A comparative study with propranolol. *J Hepatol* 1992; **15**: 48–53.

96 Hadengue A, Moreau R, Cerini R, Koshy A, Lee SS, Lebrec D. Combination of ketanserin and verapamil or propranolol in patients with alcoholic cirrhosis: search for an additive effect. *Hepatology* 1989; **9**: 83–87.

97 Pomier-Layrargues G, Giroux L, Rocheleau B, Huet PM. Combined treatment of portal hypertension with ritanserin and propranolol in conscious and unrestrained cirrhotic rats. *Hepatology* 1992; **15**: 878–882.

98 Roulot D, Gaudin C, Braillon A, Sekiyama T, Bacq Y, Lebrec D. Hemodynamic effects of combination of clonidine and propranolol in conscious cirrhotic rats. *Can J Physiol Pharmacol* 1989; **67**: 1369–1372.

99 Garcia-Pagan JC, Salmeron JM, Feu F *et al.* Spironolactone (Sp) decreases portal pressure in patients with compensated cirrhosis (abstract). *J Hepatol* 1992; **13** (Suppl. 2): S30.

100 Merkel C, Gatta A, Amodio P *et al.* Nadolol or Nadolol plus isosorbide-5-mononitrate in the prophylaxis of first variceal bleeding in patients with cirrhosis. Interim

analysis of a multicenter study. *J Hepatol* 1993; **8** (Suppl. 1): S147–S148.

101 Moreau R, Komeichi H, Cailmail S, Lebrec D. Blockade of ATP-sensitive K$^+$ channels by glibenclamide reduces portal pressure and hyperkinetic circulation in portal hypertensive rats. *J Hepatol* 1992; **16**: 215–218.

102 Moreau R, Komeichi H, Kirstetter P, Ohsuga M, Cailmail S, Lebrec D. Altered control of vascular tone by adenosinetriphosphate-sensitive potassium channels in rats with cirrhosis. *Gastroenterology* 1994; **106**: 1016–1023.

103 Standen NB, Quayle JM, Davies NW, Brayden JE, Huang Y, Nelson MT. Hyperpolarizing vasodilators activate ATP-sensitive K$^+$ channels in arterial smooth muscle. *Science* 1989; **245**: 177–180.

104 Atucha NM, Groszmann RJ. Mechanisms of vasodilation in the mesenteric vascular bed of portal hypertensive rats (abstract). *Hepatology* 1991; **20**: 100A.

105 Elkayam U. Tolerance to organic nitrates: evidence, mechanisms, clinical relevance, and strategies for prevention. *Ann Intern Med* 1991; **114**: 667–677.

106 Abrams J. Nitroglycerin and long-acting nitrates. *N Engl J Med* 1980; **302**: 1234–1237.

107 Abshagen U, Betzien G, Endele R *et al.* Pharmacokinetics of intra-venous and oral isosorbide-5- mononitrate. *Eur J Clin Pharmacol* 1981; **20**: 269–275.

108 Fung HL. Pharmacokinetics and pharmacodynamics of isosorbide dinitrate. *Am Heart J* 1985; **110**: 213–216.

109 Rector WG, Hossack KF. Vasopressin and vasopressin plus nitroglycerin for portal hypertension. Effects on systemic and splanchnic haemodynamics and coronary blood flow. *J Hepatol* 1989; **8**: 308–315.

110 Blei AT, O'Reilly DJ, Gottstein J. Portal-systemic shunting and the hemodynamic effect of nitroglycerin in the rat. *Gastroenterology* 1984; **86**: 1428–1436.

111 Kroeger RJ, Groszmann RJ. The effect of the combination of nitroglycerin and propranolol on splanchnic and systemic hemodynamics in a portal hypertensive rat model. *Hepatology* 1985; **5**: 425–430.

112 Blei AT, Gottstein J. Isosorbide dinitrate in experimental portal hypertension: a study of factors that modulate the hemodynamic response. *Hepatology* 1986; **6**: 107–111.

113 Bhathal PS, Grossmann HJ. Reduction of the increased portal vascular resistance of the isolated perfused cirrhotic rat liver by vasodilators. *J Hepatol* 1985; **1**: 325–337.

114 Marteau P, Ballet F, Chazouilleres O *et al.* Effect of vasodilators on hepatic microcirculation in cirrhosis: a study in the isolated perfused rat liver. *Hepatology* 1989; **9**: 820–823.

115 Hallemans R, Naeije R, Mols P, Melot C, Reding P. Treatment of portal hypertension with isosorbide dinitrate alone and in combination with vasopressin *Crit Care Med* 1983; **11**: 536–540.

116 Freeman JG, Barton JR, Record CO. Effect of isosorbide dinitrate, verapamil and labetalol on portal pressure in cirrhosis. *Br Med J* 1985; **291**: 752–755.

117 Garcia-Tsao G, Groszmann RJ. Portal hemodynamics during nitroglycerin administration in cirrhotic patients. *Hepatology* 1987; **7**: 805–809.

118 Merkel C, Finucci G, Zuin R *et al.* Effects of isosorbide dinitrate on portal hypertension in alcoholic patients. *J Hepatol* 1987; **4**: 174–180.

119 Blei AT, Garcia-Tsao G, Groszmann RJ. Hemodynamic evaluation of isosorbide dinitrate in alcoholic cirrhosis. Pharmacokinetic–hemodynamic interactions. *Gastroenterology* 1987; **93**: 576–583.

120 Westaby D, Gimson AES, Hayes PC *et al.* Haemodynamic response to intravenous vasopressin and nitroglycerin in portal hypertension. *Gut* 1988; **29**: 372–377.

121 Hayes PC, Westaby D, Williams R. Effect and mechanism of action of isosorbide-5-mononitrate. *Gut* 1988; **29**: 752–755.

122 Mols P, Hallemans R, Melot C, Lejeune P, Naeije R. Systemic and regional hemodynamic effects of isosorbide dinitrate in patients with liver cirrhosis and portal hypertension. *J Hepatol* 1989; **8**: 316–324.

123 Navasa M, Chesta J, Bosch J, Rodes J. Reduction of portal pressure by isosorbide-5-mononitrate in patients with cirrhosis. Effects on splanchnic and systemic hemodynamics and liver function. *Gastroenterology* 1989; **96**: 1110–1118.

124 Garcia-Pagan JC, Feu F, Navasa M *et al.* Long-term haemodynamic effects of isosorbide-5-mononitrate in patients with cirrhosis and portal hypertension. *J Hepatol* 1990; **11**: 189–195.

125 Iwao T, Toyonaga A, Sumino M *et al.* Hemodynamic study during transdermal application of nitroglycerin tape in patients with cirrhosis. *Hepatology* 1991; **13**: 124–128.

126 Grose RD, Plevris JN, Rehead DN, Bouchier IAD, Hayes PC. The acute and chronic effects of isosorbide-5-mononitrate on portal haemodynamics in cirrhosis. *J Hepatol* 1994; **20**: 542–547.

127 Noguchi H, Toyonaga A, Tanikawa K. Influence of nitroglycerin on portal pressure and gastric mucosal hemodynamics in patients with cirrhosis. *J Gastroenterol* 1994; **29**: 180–188.

128 Ikegami M, Toyonaga A, Tanikawa K. Reduction of portal pressure by chronic administration of isosorbide dinitrate in patients with cirrhosis: effects on systemic and splanchnic haemodynamics and liver function. *Am J Gastroenterol* 1992; **87**: 1160–1164.

129 Vorobioff J, Picabea E, Gamen M, Villavicencio R. Isosorbide dinitrate in portal hypertensive patients. *J Hepatol* 1992; **16**: 387.

130 Salmeron JM, Ruiz del Arbol L, Gines A *et al.* Renal effects of acute isosorbide-5-mononitrate administration in cirrhosis. *Hepatology* 1993; **17**: 800–806.

131 Atkinson M. The effect of diuretics on portal pressure. *Lancet* 1959; **ii**: 819–823.

132 Weisberg H, Rosenthal WS, Glass GBJ. The effect of diuretic therapy on portal pressure in cirrhotic patients with and without ascites. *Am J Dig Dis* 1965; **10**: 293–299.

133 Cereda J-M, Roulot D, Braillon A, Moreaus R, Koshy A, Lebrec D. Reduction of portal pressure by acute administration of furosemide in patients with alcoholic cirrhosis. *J Hepatol* 1989; **9**: 246–251.

134 Okumura H, Arakami T, Katsuta Y *et al.* Reduction in hepatic venous pressure gradient as a consequence of volume contraction due to chronic administration of spironolactone in patients with cirrhosis and no ascites. *Am J Gastroenterol* 1991; **86**: 46–52.

135 Bertoni G, Sassatelli R, Fornaciari G *et al.* Oral isosorbide-5-mononitrate reduces the rebleeding rate during the course of injection sclerotherapy for esophageal varices. *Scand J Gastroenterol* 1994; **29**: 363–370.

136 Villanueva C, Balanzo J, Novella MT. A prospective and randomized trial of endoscopic sclerotherapy (es) vs nadolol plus isosorbide-5-mononitrate (Is-5-Mn) for the prevention of variceal rebleeding (abstract). *Hepatology* 1994; **20**: 268A.

137 Vinel J-P, Monnin J-L, Combis J- M, Cales P, Desmorat H, Pascal J-P. Hemodynamic evaluation of molsidomine: a vasodilator with antianginal properties in patients with alcoholic cirrhosis. *Hepatology* 1990; **11**: 239–242.

138 Kukovetz WR, Holzmann S. Mechanism of vasodilation by molsidomine. *Am Heart J* 1985; **109**: 637–640.

139 Takeshita A, Nakamura M, Tajimi T *et al.* Long lasting effect of oral molsidomine on exercise performance: a new antianginal agent. *Circulation* 1977; **55**: 401–07.

140 Majid PA, De Feyter PJF, Van Der Wall EE, Wardeh R, Roos J-P. Molsidomine in the treatment of patients with angina pectoris: acute hemodynamic effects and clinical efficacy. *N Engl J Med* 1980; **302**: 1–6.

141 Stewart DJ, Elsner D, Sommer O, Holtz J, Bassenge E. Altered spectrum of nitroglycerin-specific venous tolerance with maintenance of arterial vasodepressor potency. *Circulation* 1986; **74**: 573–582.

142 Ruiz del Arbol L, Garcia-Pagan JC, Feu F, Pizcueta MP, Bosch J, Rodes J. Effects of molsidomine, a long acting venous dilator, on portal hypertension. A hemodynamic study in patients with cirrhosis. *J Hepatol* 1991; **13**(2): 179–186.

143 Monnin J-L, Vinel J-P, Pascal J-P *et al.* Pulsed doppler flowmetry assessment of molsidomine and molsidomine + propranolol effects on portal hemodynamics in patients with cirrhosis. *Gastroenterol Clin Biol* 1991; **16**(10): 745–750.

144 Desmorat H, Vinel J-P, Lahlou O *et al.* Systemic and splanchnic hemodynamic effects of molsidomine in rats with carbon tetrachloride-induced cirrhosis. *Hepatology* 1991; **13**: 1181–1184.

145 Huppe D, Jager D, Tromm A, Tunn S, Barmeyer J, May B. Acute and long term effects of molsidomine on portal and cardiac hemodynamics in patients with cirrhosis of the liver. *Eur J Gastroenterol Hepatol* 1992; **4**: 849–855.

146 van Zwieten PA, Timmermans PBMWM. Pharmacology and characterization of central alpha-adrenoreceptors involved in the effect of centrally acting antihypertensive drugs. *Chest* 1983; **83**: 340–343.

147 Roulot D, Braillon A, Gaudin C, Ozier Y, Girod C, Lebrec D. Mechanisms of a clonidine-induced decrease in portal pressure in normal and cirrhotic conscious rats. *Hepatology* 1989; **10**: 477–481.

148 Willet IR, Esler M, Jennings G, Dudley FJ. Sympathetic tone modulate portal venous pressure in alcoholic cirrhosis. *Lancet* 1986; **2**: 939–943.

149 Moreau R, Lee SS, Hadengue A, Braillon A, Lebrec D. Hemodynamic effects of a clonidine-induced decrease in sympathetic tone in patients with cirrhosis. *Hepatology* 1987; **7**: 147–154.

150 Roulot D, Moreau R, Gaudin C *et al.* Long-term sympathetic and hemodynamic responses to clonidine in patients with cirrhosis and ascites. *Gastroenterology* 1992; **102**: 1309–1318.

151 Esler M, Dudley F, Jennings G *et al.* Increased sympathetic nervous activity and the effects of its inhibition with clonidine in alcoholic cirrhosis. *Ann Intern Med* 1992; **116**: 446–455.

152 Albillos A, Banares R, Barrios C *et al.* Oral administration of clonidine in patients with alcoholic cirrhosis. *Gastroenterology* 1992; **102**: 248–254.

153 Roulot D, Moreau R, Gaudin C *et al.* Long-term beneficial effects of clonidine on renal and splanchnic hemodynamics in patients with cirrhosis and ascites (abstract). *Hepatology* 1989; **10**: 589.

154 Cummings SA, Groszmann RJ, Kaumann AJ. Hypersensitivity of mesenteric veins to 5-hydroxytryptamine- and ketanserin-induced reduction of portal pressure in portal hypertensive rats. *Br J Pharmacol* 1986; **89**: 501–513.

155 Cummings SA, Kaumann AJ, Groszmann RJ. Comparison of the hemodynamic responses to ketanserin and prazosin in portal hypertensive rats. *Hepatology* 1988; **8**: 1112–1115.

156 Mastai R, Brault A, Huet P-M. Effects of serotonin on the microcirculation of the normal perfused rat liver (abstract). *Hepatology* 1987; **7**: 1032.

157 Richardson PDI, Withrington PG. A comparison of the effects of bradykinin, 5-hydroxytryptamine and histamine on the hepatic arterial and portal venous vascular beds in the dog: histamine H1 and H2 receptor populations. *Br J Pharmacol* 1977; **60**: 123–133.

158 Hadengue A, Lee SS, Moreau R, Braillon A, Lebrec D. Beneficial hemodynamic effects of ketanserin in patients with cirrhosis: possible role of serotonergic mechanisms in portal hypertension. *Hepatology* 1987; **7**: 644–647.

159 Vorobioff J, Garcia-Tsao G, Groszmann RJ et al. Long-term hemodynamic effects of ketanserin, a 5-hydroxytryptamine blocker, in portal hypertensive patients. *Hepatology* 1989; **9**: 88–91.

160 Hadengue A, Moreau R, Cerini R, Koshy A, Lee SS, Lebrec D. Combination of ketanserin and verapamil or propranolol in patients with alcoholic cirrhosis: search for an additive effect. *Hepatology* 1989; **9**: 83–87.

161 Lee F-Y, Tsai Y-T, Lin H-C et al. Hemodynamic effects of a combination of vasopressin and ketanserin in patients with hepatitis B-related cirrhosis. *J Hepatol* 1992; **15**: 54–58.

162 Leysen JE, Gommeren W, Van Gompel P et al. Receptor-binding properties *in vitro* and *in vivo* of ritanserin: a very potent and long acting serotonin-S2 antagonist. *Mol Pharmacol* 1985; **27**: 600–611.

163 Gradin K, Pettersson A, Persson B. Chronic 5HT2-receptor blockade with ritanserin does not reduce the blood pressure in the spontaneously hypertensive rats. *J Neural Transm* 1985; **64**: 145–149.

164 Mastai R, Rocheleau B, Huet P-M. Serotonin blockade in conscious, unrestrained cirrhotic dogs with portal hypertension. *Hepatology* 1989; **9**: 265–268.

165 Mastai R, Giroux L, Semret M, Huet P-M. Ritanserin decreases portal pressure in conscious and unrestrained cirrhotic rats. *Gastroenterology* 1990; **98**: 141–145.

166 Nevens F, Pizcueta M, Fernandez M, Bosch J, Rodes J. Effects of ritanserin, a selective and specific S2-serotonergic antagonist, on portal pressure and splanchnic hemodynamics in portal hypertensive rats. *Hepatology* 1991; **14**: 1174–1178.

167 Fernandez M, Pizcueta P, Garcia-Pagan JC et al. Effects of ritanserin, a selective and specific S2-serotonergic antagonist, on portal pressure and splanchnic hemodynamics in rats with long-term bile duct ligation. *Hepatology* 1993; **18**: 389–393.

168 Huet P-M, Pomier-Layrargues G, Semret M. Effects of ritanserin, a serotonin antagonist, in cirrhotic patients with portal hypertension (abstract). *Hepatology* 1988; **8**: 1422.

169 Pomier-Layrargues G, Giroux L, Rochleau B, Huet P-M. Combined treatment of portal hypertension with ritanserin and propranolol in conscious and unrestrained cirrhotic rats. *Hepatology* 1992; **15**: 878–882.

170 Mills PR, Rae AP, Farah DA, Russell RI, Lorimer AR, Carter DC. Comparison of three adrenoreceptor blocking agents in patients with cirrhosis and portal hypertension. *Gut* 1984; **25**: 73–78.

171 Albillos A, Lledo JL, Banares R et al. Hemodynamic effects of alpha-adrenergic blockade with prazosin in cirrhotic patients with portal hypertension. *Hepatology* 1994; **20**: 611–617.

172 Reichen J, Le M. Verapamil favourably influences hepatic microvascular exchange and function in rats with cirrhosis of the liver. *J Clin Invest* 1986; **78**: 448–455.

173 Reichen J, Hirlinger A, Ha HR, Sagesser S. Chronic verapamil administration lowers

portal pressure and improves hepatic function in rats with liver cirrhosis. *J Hepatol* 1986; **3**: 49–58.

174 Kong C-W, Lay C-S, Tsai Y-T *et al.* The hemodynamic effect of verapamil on portal hypertension in patients with postnecrotic cirrhosis. *Hepatology* 1986; **6**: 423–426.

175 Boyer TD, Trigger DR, Horisawa M, Redeker AG, Reynolds TB. Direct transhepatic measurement of portal vein pressure using a thin needle. Comparison with wedged hepatic vein pressure. *Gastroenterology* 1977; **72**: 584–589.

176 Pomier-Layrargues G, Kusielewicz D, Willems B *et al.* Presinusoidal portal hypertension in non-alcoholic cirrhosis. *Hepatology* 1985; **5**: 415–418.

177 Lin H-C, Tsai Y-T, Lee F-Y *et al.* Comparison between portal vein pressure and wedged hepatic vein pressure in hepatitis B-related cirrhosis. *J Hepatol* 1989; **9**: 326–330.

178 Iwao T, Toyonaga A, Ikegami M *et al.* Wedged hepatic venous pressure reflects portal venous pressure during vasoactive drug administration in nonalcoholic cirrhosis. *Dig Dis Sci* 1994; **39**: 2439–2444.

179 Vinel JP, Caucanas JB, Cales P *et al.* Effects of verapamil on portohepatic gradient and metabolic activity of the liver in alcoholic cirrhosis (abstract). *J Hepatol* 1987; **5** (Suppl. 1): S221.

180 Merkel C, Finucci GF, Bolognesi M *et al.* The calcium-channel blocker, verapamil, does not improve portal pressure of liver metabolic activity in alcoholic cirrhosis (abstract). *J Hepatol* 1987; **6** (Suppl. 1): S168.

181 Navasa M, Bosch J, Reichen J *et al.* Effects of verapamil on hepatic and systemic hemodynamics and liver function in patients with cirrhosis and portal hypertension. *Hepatology* 1988; **8**: 850–854.

182 Koshy A, Hadengue A, Lee SS *et al.* Possible deleterious hemodynamic effect of nifedipine on portal hypertension in patients with cirrhosis. *Clin Pharmacol Ther* 1987; **42**: 295–298.

183 Iwao T, Toyonaga A, Ikegami M *et al.* Nicardipine infusion improved hepatic function but failed to reduce hepatic venous pressure gradient in patients with cirrhosis. *Am J Gastroenterol* 1992; **87**: 326–331.

184 Iwao T, Toyonaga A, Ikegami M *et al.* Effects of vasopressin and nicardipine on hemodynamics and liver function in patients with cirrhosis: comparison with vasopressin alone. *J Hepatol* 1993; **19**: 345–352.

185 Garcia-Pagan JC, Feu F, Luca A *et al.* Nicardipine increases hepatic blood flow and the hepatic clearance of indocyanine green in patients with cirrhosis. *J Hepatol* 1994; **20**: 792–796.

186 Miskowiak J. How the lower oesophageal sphincter affects submucosal oesophageal varices. *Lancet* 1978; **ii**: 1284–1285.

187 Miskowiak J, Burcharth F, Jensen LI. Effect of lower oesophageal sphincter on oesophageal varices. A portographic study. *Scand J Gastroenterol* 1981; **16**: 957–960.

188 Lunderquist A, Alwmark A, Gullstrand P *et al.* Pharmacologic influence on esophageal varices: a preliminary report. *Cardiovascular Intervent Radiol* 1983; **6**: 65–71.

189 Owman T, Lunderquist A. Pharmacologic manipulation of lower esophageal sphincter pressure. A possible means of treatment of variceal bleeding. *Radiologie* 1983; **23**: 139–142.

190 Mastai R, Grande L, Bosch J *et al.* Effects of metoclopramide and domperidone on azygous venous blood flow in patients with cirrhosis and portal hypertension. *Hepatology* 1986; **6**: 1244–1247.

191 Braillon A, Capron-Chivrac D, Valla D, Lee SS, Capron J-P, Lebrec D. Domperidone-induced increase in lower oesophageal sphincter pressure does not affect azygous blood flow in patients with cirrhosis. *Scand J Gastroenterol* 1986; **21**: 1080–1082.

192 Hoevels J. Does domperidone modify the hemodynamics of esophageal varices? R O F O: *Fortschritte auf dem Gabiete der Rontgenstrahlen und der Niklearmedizin* 1989; **150**: 462–464.

193 Taranto D, Suozzo R, de Sio I *et al.* Effect of metoclopramide on transmural oeso-phageal variceal pressure and portal blood flow in cirrhotic patients. *Digestion* 1990; **47**: 56–60.

194 Stanciu C, Cijevschi C, Stan M, Sandulescu E. Endoscopic intravascular esophageal pressure measurements in cirrhotic patients: response to metoclopramide. *Hepato-Gastroenterology* 1993; **40**: 173–175.

195 Kleber G, Sauerbruch T, Fischer G, Geigenberger G, Paumgartner G. Reduction of transmural oesophageal variceal pressure by metoclopramide. *J Hepatol* 1991; **12**: 362–366

196 Saraya A, Sarin SK. Effects of intravenous nitroglycerin and metoclopramide on intravariceal pressure: a double-blind, randomized study. *Am J Gastroenterol* 1993; **8** 1850–1853.

197 Ljubicic N. Effect of metoclopramide on portal blood flow in patients with liver cirrhosis, measured by the pulsed Doppler system. *Scand J Gastroenterol* 1990; **25**: 1004–1009.

198 Hosking SW, Doss W, El-Zeiny H, Robinson P, Barsoum MS, Johnson AG. Phar-macological constriction of the lower oesophageal sphincter: a simple method of arresting variceal haemorrhage. *Gut* 1988; **29**: 1098–1102.

199 Gupta IP, Sharma MP. Control of variceal bleed with metoclopramide. *Ind J Gas-troenterol* 1991; **10**: 10–11.

200 Feu F, Mas A, Bosch J *et al.* Domperidone or metoclopramide vs placebo in the prevention of early variceal rebleeding in cirrhosis. A prospective, randomized trial (abstract). *J Hepatol* 1988; **7**: S31.

201 Ohta M, Hashizume M, Tanoue K *et al.* Metoclopramide inhibits development of esophageal varices in rat model. *Dig Dis Sci* 1994; **39**: 1853–1858.

202 Carey RM, Thorner MO, Ortt EM. Effects of metoclopramide and bromocriptine on the renin-angiotensin-aldosterone system in man: dopaminergic control of aldoster-one. *J Clin Invest* 1979; **63**: 727–735.

203 Sowers JR, Sharp B, McCallum RW. Effect of domperidone, an extracerebral inhi-bitor of dopamine receptor, on thyrotropin, prolactin, renin, aldosterone and 18-hydroxycorticosterone secretion in man. *J Clin Endocrinol Metab* 1982; **54**: 869–871.

204 D'Arienzo A, Ambrogio G, Di Siervi P, Perna E, Squame G, Mazzacca G. A rando-mized comparison of metoclopramide and domperidone on plasma aldosterone concentration and on spironolactone-induced diuresis in ascitic cirrhotic patients. *Hepatology* 1985; **5**: 854–857.

205 Gholson CF, Freeman MR. Letter. *Hepatology* 1987; **7**: 800.

206 Albillos A, Colombato LA, Groszmann RJ. Vasodilatation and sodium retention in prehepatic portal hypertension. *Gastroenterology* 1992; **102**: 931–935.

207 Colombato LA, Albillos A, Groszmann RJ. Temporal relationship of peripheral vasodilatation, plasma volume expansion and the hyperdynamic circulatory state in portal hypertensive rats. *Hepatology* 1992; **15**: 323–328.

208 Schrier RW, Arroyo V, Bernardi M, Epstein M, Henriksen JH, Rodes J. Peripheral

arterial vasodilatation hypothesis: a proposal for the initiation of renal sodium and water retention. *Hepatology* 1988; **8**: 1151–1157.

209 Atkinson M. The effect of diuretics on portal venous pressure. *Lancet* 1959; ii: 819–823.

210 Weisberg H, Rosenthal WS, Glass GBJ. The effect of diuretic therapy on portal pressure in cirrhotic patients with and without ascites. *Am J Dig Dis* 1965; **10**: 293–299.

211 Cereda J-M, Roulot D, Braillon A, Moreau R, Koshy A, Lebrec D. Reduction of portal pressure by acute administration of furosemide in patients with alcoholic cirrhosis. *J Hepatol* 1989; **9**: 246–251.

212 Okumura H, Arakami T, Katsuta Y *et al.* Reduction in hepatic venous pressure gradient as a consequence of volume contraction due to chronic administration of spironolactone in patients with cirrhosis and no ascites. *Am J Gastroenterol* 1991; **86**: 46–52.

213 Genecin P, Polio J, Groszmann RJ. Na restriction blunts expansion of plasma volume and ameliorates hyperdynamic circulation in portal hypertension. *Am J Physiol* 1990; **259**: G498–G503.

214 Garcia-Pagan JC, Salmeron JM, Feu F *et al.* Effects of low-sodium diet and spironolactone on portal pressure in patients with compensated cirrhosis. *Hepatology* 1994; **19**: 1095–1099.

215 Sogni P, Soupison T, Moreau R *et al.* Hemodynamic effects of acute administration of furosemide in patients with cirrhosis receiving beta-adrenergic antagonists *J Hepatol* 1994; **20**: 548–552.

216 Katsuta Y, Aramaki T, Sekiyama T, Satomura K, Okumura K. Plasma volume contraction in portal hypertension. *J Hepatol* 1993; **17** (Suppl. 2): S19–S23.

217 Garcia-Pagan JC, Salmeron JM, Feu F *et al.* Spironolactone (Sp) decreases portal pressure in patients with compensated cirrhosis (abstract). *J Hepatol* 1991; **13** (Suppl. 2): S30.

Baveno II Consensus Statements: Drug Therapy for Portal Hypertension

Roberto J. Groszmann (Chairman), Flemming Bendtsen, Jaime Bosch, Wolfgang Fleig, Norman Grace, Didier Lebrec, Carlo Merkel and Jean Pierre Vinel

1   The most remarkable advances of the past 5 years on drug therapy for portal hypertension are:

(a) general acceptance of pharmacological therapy as an important option in the treatment of portal hypertension;

(b) some important advances which have been made in the basic understanding of portal hypertension may be the basis for further progress in this area.

2   For prophylactic treatment with pharmacological agents:

(a) at the present time the data support the treatment of patients with large varices; however, studies are on the way to evaluate the usefulness of pharmacological therapy in the treatment of small varices.

3   At the present time, the drug(s) of choice for the prevention of the first variceal bleeding are:

(a) non-selective beta-adrenergic blockers;

(b) isosorbide-5-mononitrate, which might be prescribed in case of intolerance or contraindications to beta-blockers.

4   The HVPG is an extremely useful technique for the management of patients with portal hypertension as:

(a) it may be recommended for prophylactic treatment of the first variceal haemorrhage;

(b) its use is strongly recommended in patients that are being treated for the prevention of rebleeding. In this respect, it should be used as the 'gold standard'.

5   For treatment of acute variceal bleeding:

(a) glypressin is effective and has been shown to improve survival;

(b) somatostatin has been shown to be as effective as other comparable therapies;

(c) insufficient data are available with octreotide;

(d) vasopressin should be used only in conjunction with NTG.

6   Combination of drugs to prevent first bleeding and rebleeding:

(a) insufficient information is available. However, the time has probably come to use combinations for these indications. This is certainly an area that will benefit from new trials.

7 For prevention of rebleeding:
   (a) if there are no contraindications, the association of beta-blockers and sclerotherapy could be used to prevent rebleeding.
8 For treatment of portal hypertensive gastropathy:
   (a) only patients with severe gastropathy and bleeding should be treated with portal pressure-reducing agents;
   (b) drug combinations are being tested.

A Look into the Future of the Pharmacological Treatment of Portal Hypertension

Didier Lebrec and Richard Moreau

INTRODUCTION

Gastrointestinal bleeding due to ruptured varices occurs in patients with collateral circulation which is a result of portal hypertension. The pharmacological treatment of portal hypertension consists of decreasing portal pressure and reducing the risk of its complications. In patients with chronic liver disease, elevated portal pressure mainly depends on extensive fibrosis (Fig. 4). Thus, the best treatment for portal hypertension is to prevent the development of hepatic fibrosis and cirrhosis. In patients with portal hypertension, the prevention of the development of superior portosystemic shunts and varices is the best treatment to prevent gastrointestinal bleeding. Finally, when oesophageal varices are present, certain vasoactive substances may reduce the risk of bleeding by decreasing portal blood flow or intrahepatic vascular resistance. Most of these drugs increase intracellular calcium levels (see below). This chapter reviews various new approaches to the pharmacological treatment of portal hypertension.

PREVENTION OF CHRONIC LIVER DISEASE AND HEPATIC FIBROSIS

Certain liver diseases may be prevented by abstinence from alcohol, by education in endemic areas of *Schistosoma mansoni* and by vaccination against hepatitis viruses, while others should be treated to prevent the development of chronic liver diseases and hepatic fibrosis. Hepatic fibrosis may be prevented by eliminating the specific fibrogenic stimuli. For example, the copper overload in Wilson's disease and the iron overload in haemochromatosis are both treated with chelation therapy. Alpha-interferon has been shown to decrease fibrogenesis in patients with chronic hepatitis B or C. Anti-schistosomal treatment prevents the fibrinogenesis of schistosomiasis. Finally, although discontinuing alcohol may prevent cirrhosis, different substances have also been proposed whose efficacy must still be demonstrated (Table 10).

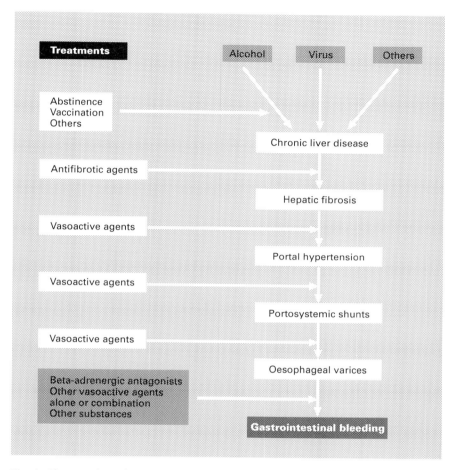

Fig. 4. Pharmacological prevention and treatment of portal hypertension.

Table 10 Pharmacological treatment of alcohol-induced hepatic toxicity.

Colchicine
Phosphatidylcholine
Propylthiouracyl
S-adenosylmethionine
Steroids

In chronic liver disease, fibrogenic stimuli cannot be removed and fibrosis is already present. In this case, the inhibition of hepatic fibrogenesis is necessary [1,2]. Treatment of hepatic fibrosis can be classified into the following groups: hepatoprotectors, anti-inflammatory and immunosuppressors, antifibrogenic and collagenase inducers (Table 11).

Table 11 Pharmacological agents that may limit hepatic fibrogenesis.

Treatment types	Drugs
Hepatoprotector	Malotilate Prostaglandins Ursodeoxycholic acid Silymarin
Anti-inflammatory and immunosupressor	Colchicine Cyclosporin Methotrexate Progesterone Steroids
Antifibrogenic	D-penicillamine Lysyloxidase inhibitor Oxoglutarate inibiitor Pentoxifylline Proline analogue Prolyl-4-hydroxylase inhibitor
Collagenase inducer	Polyunsaturated lecithin
Others	Collagen propeptides Decorin γ-Interferon Glucocorticoid Retinoid

Hepatoprotector agents mainly prevent cell damage, decrease the production of colony stimulating factors, and diminish the number of inflammatory cells. Other mechanisms can, however, be implicated, for example by decreasing collagen deposition. The administration of ursodedeoxycholic acid reduces the toxic effects of the more hydrophobic bile acids and thus has a beneficial effect. The efficacy of hepatoprotector agents has been demonstrated in certain models of cirrhosis while clinical studies have shown that this type of drug limits the development of liver disease.

Inflammation is a component which precedes and accompanies fibrogenesis and may activate collagen-producing cells, while anti-inflammatory drugs may play a role in the prevention of hepatic fibrosis and portal hypertension. Experimental studies have shown an efficacy, while discrepant results were observed in clinical studies.

The prevention of collagen accumulation would be the ideal treatment of portal hypertension in patients with cirrhosis. The mechanisms involved in the regulation of collagen gene expression have not yet been determined. Each stage requires a specific enzyme which could be a target for pharmacological treatment. In fact, a drug may modify only one stage of the biosynthetic pathway and thus, several agents may be necessary. More experimental and clinical studies are needed. Finally, *in vitro* studies have shown that certain substances induce collagenase activity or production in various cultured mesenchymal cells.

PREVENTION OF PORTOSYSTEMIC SHUNTS AND VARICES

Different experimental studies have evaluated the prevention of portal hypertension and portosystemic shunts by early chronic administration of vasoactive substances in animals with portal hypertension [3–5]. In rats with portal vein stenosis, clonidine or propranolol were administered 3 days before portal vein stenosis and then administered continuously for 10 consecutive days [3,4]. In treated rats, both portal pressure and mesenteric–systemic shunts were significantly lower than in the placebo group. Similar results were observed in a chronic murine schistosomiasis model [5]. These studies showed that early administration of beta-adrenergic antagonists or a centrally acting alpha$_2$-adrenergic agonist limit the severity of portal hypertension and the development of portosystemic shunts in portal hypertensive animals. These beneficial effects were probably due to a limitation of the initial increase in portal pressure.

Two clinical studies have been performed to evaluate the effect and safety of long-acting propranolol in unselected patients with mild or moderate chronic liver disease resulting from different causes [6,7]. In a first 1-year study, none of the 47 patients in the propranolol group bled compared with three of 48 patients given placebo. In another study, propranolol was administered to unselected patients with chronic liver disease to prevent variceal bleeding. There were no statistical differences between the two groups for variceal bleeding and death. The low bleeding event rates observed in these unselected patients might explain the lack of difference between the two groups. Further clinical studies are needed to evaluate the development of oesophageal varices rather than the risk of bleeding in unselected patients with chronic liver disease.

PREVENTION OF GASTROINTESTINAL BLEEDING

The efficacy of beta-adrenergic antagonists on the risk of bleeding or rebleeding and death has been well demonstrated [8]. This type of drug, however, is either contraindicated or ineffective in certain patients. Thus, vasoactive substances other than beta-blockers (Table 12) or a combination of substances with beta-blockers (Table 13) must be proposed for the pharmacological treatment of portal hypertension.

Table 12 Drugs that cause a long-term decrease in portal hypertension in patients with cirrhosis.

Type	Drugs
Alpha-adrenergic antagonist	Prazosin
Alpha$_2$-adrenergic agonist	Clonidine
Beta-adrenergic antagonist	
Non-selective	Long-acting propranolol
	Nadolol
	Propranolol
Cardioselective	Atenolol
Diuretic	Chlorothiazide
	Spironolactone
5-HT$_2$ receptor antagonist	Ketanserin
	Ritanserin
Nitrovasodilator	Isosorbide-5-mononitrate
	Isosorbide dinitrate
	Molsidomine

Table 13 Drugs combined with propranolol that cause a further decrease in portal hypertension.

Type	Drugs
Alpha$_2$-adrenergic agonist	Clonidine
Diuretic	Spironolactone
5-HT$_2$ receptor antagonist	Ketanserin
	Ritanserin
Nitrovasodilator	Isosorbide-5-mononitrate
	Molsidomine
	Nipradilol

Apart from non-selective beta-adrenergic antagonists, some vasoactive substances continuously decrease portal pressure in patients with portal hypertension [8].

Alpha-adrenergic antagonists

One clinical study showed that chronic administration of prasozin induced a sustained 20% decrease in the hepatic venous pressure gradient in patients with cirrhosis [9]. No significant change was observed in the systemic circulation.

Alpha$_2$-adrenergic agonists

In cirrhosis, clonidine, a centrally acting alpha$_2$-agonist has been shown to decrease the elevated sympathetic nervous activity which plays a role in the production of portal hypertension. Thus, clonidine has been used to reduce the degree of portal hypertension. Two clinical studies evaluated the long-term haemodynamic effects of clonidine in patients with cirrhosis [10,11]. Clonidine administration decreased both plasma noradrenaline concentrations and the hepatic venous pressure gradient, while hepatic blood flow was not affected. Clonidine also caused a mild decrease in arterial pressure and cardiac output which was well tolerated. During long-term treatment, liver tests and intrinsic hepatic clearance were not altered.

Diuretics

Since patients with portal hypertension have elevated blood volume, diuretics have been used to reduce the degree of portal hypertension through a reduction of blood volume. Three clinical studies have evaluated the long-term effects of diuretics [12–14]. All these studies showed that chronic administration of diuretics significantly decreased portal pressure estimated by the hepatic venous pressure gradient or splenic pulp pressure. The reduction in portal pressure was associated with a significant decrease in blood volume. Long-term administration of diuretics also significantly reduced both arterial pressure and cardiac output. No side effects were observed.

Five-hydroxytryptamine (5-HT$_2$) receptor antagonists

Two clinical studies evaluated the long-term haemodynamic effects of 5-HT$_2$ receptor antagonists; one used ritanserin [15] and the other ketanserin [16]. The first study with eight patients showed that continuous administration of ritanserin caused a significant decrease in the hepatic venous pressure gradient with no systemic haemodynamic effects. Ritanserin was well tolerated in all patients. The second study showed that ketanserin significantly decreased the hepatic venous pressure gradient as well as cardiac output and arterial pressure. Mild and reversible hepatic encephalopathy occurred, however, in some patients with severe liver disease.

Nitrovasodilators

Five studies have tested three different nitrovasodilators for a long period in patients with cirrhosis [17–21]. These investigations showed that isosorbide-

5-mononitrate or isosorbide dinitrate and molsidomine reduced the hepatic venous pressure gradient to an extent ranging from 7 to 44%. The study of the systemic haemodynamic effects of nitrovasodilators showed that high doses induced a marked reduction in arterial pressure; this reduction was less marked than that observed after short-term administration.

One clinical trial compared the effects of propranolol and isosorbide-5-mononitrate on the prevention of first bleeding in patients with cirrhosis [22]. The preliminary results showed that at 2 years, the risk of bleeding and the survival rate were not significantly different between the two groups, although these need to be confirmed.

Combination of drugs

Beta-blocker and vasodilator

Since beta-blockers decrease portal pressure by reducing portal tributary blood flow and nitrovasodilators by reducing hepatic vascular resistance, a combination of propranolol and isosorbide-5-mononitrate has been tested in patients with cirrhosis [23,24]. In one study, the administration of isosorbide-5-mononitrate in patients receiving propranolol caused a further decrease in the hepatic venous pressure gradient without changing the azygos blood flow. Arterial pressure also decreased [23]. The combination of propranolol and molsidomine showed a greater reduction in portal blood flow measured by echo–Doppler than with propranolol or molsidomine alone [24]. The long-term effect of propranolol plus isosorbide-5-mono-nitrate has also been studied in patients with cirrhosis [25]. Finally, nipra-dilol, a new beta-adrenergic antagonist, combined with a nitroxy-base has been tested in patients with portal hypertension [26]. The long-term hae-modynamic effects of nipradilol on the hepatic venous pressure gradient were similar to those of propranolol alone.

Beta-blocker and 5-hydroxytryptamine receptor antagonist

In patients with cirrhosis who were receiving propranolol, the addition of ketanserin induced a further significant reduction in the hepatic venous pressure gradient and azygos blood flow [27]. Among the non-responders to propranolol, certain patients have a reduced wedged hepatic venous pressure after the addition of ketanserin. The combination of propranolol and ritanserin has been studied in conscious rats with cirrhosis [28]. This experimental study showed that the combination had more pronounced effects on portal pressure than propranolol or ketanserin alone.

Beta-blocker and alpha$_2$-adrenergic agonist

In rats with cirrhosis, it has been shown that the combination of propranolol and clonidine had a more marked effect on portal pressure and portal tributary blood flow than propranolol or clonidine alone [29]. In this study, arterial pressure was not affected but the decrease in cardiac output was more marked following the combination than with propranolol or clonidine alone.

Beta-blocker and diuretic

Preliminary results showed that the addition of propranolol in patients receiving spironolactone caused a further decrease in the hepatic venous pressure gradient [30]. This finding was not observed with the addition of furosemide in patients receiving propranolol [31].

MOLECULAR MECHANISMS FOR THE TREATMENT OF PORTAL HYPERTENSION

In arterial smooth-muscle cells, changes in cytosolic free calcium (Ca^{2+}) concentrations ($[Ca^{2+}]_i$) are responsible for variations in muscular tone. Increased $[Ca^{2+}]_i$ induces vasoconstriction while decreased $[Ca^{2+}]_i$ leads to vasorelaxation. In cirrhosis, a decrease in $[Ca^{2+}]_i$ contributes to vasodilatation. This decrease occurs by at least three different mechanisms: activation of the nitric oxide (NO)/cyclic guanosine monophosphate (cGMP) pathway, activation of the cyclic adenosine monophosphate (cAMP) pathway, and opening of potassium (K^+) channels.

The first mechanism for cirrhosis-induced reduction in $[Ca^{2+}]_i$ is the overproduction of NO by shear stress (due to high blood flow) and increased production of neuropeptides (substance P, calcitonin gene-related peptide (CGRP), vasoactive intestinal peptide (VIP)) [32–34]. All these factors stimulate the enzyme NO-synthase to produce NO [35]. In arterial smooth-muscle cells, NO stimulates a soluble guanylyl cyclase to produce the cyclic nucleotide, cGMP. This activates cGMP-dependent protein kinase (or cGMP-kinase) which induces a reduction in $[Ca^{2+}]_i$ [36].

The second mechanism for $[Ca^{2+}]_i$ reduction is the increase in concentrations of certain substances such as PGI_2, glucagon, neuropeptides (CGRP and VIP) and beta$_2$-adrenoceptor agonists, at the level of arterial smooth-muscle cells. These substances stimulate the production of another cyclic nucleotide, cAMP, in arterial smooth-muscle cells [36]. Cyclic adenosine monophosphate has been shown to induce a reduction in $[Ca^{2+}]_i$ (and a subsequent vasorelaxation) by activating cGMP-kinase [37,38]. This kinase, therefore, is the common final pathway by which two main cyclic nucleotides, cGMP and cAMP, decrease vascular tone in cirrhosis (Fig. 5) [36].

Cyclic guanosine monophospate-dependent protein kinase may decrease $[Ca^{2+}]_i$ by at least three different mechanisms. First, the stimulation of Ca^{2+} pumps located in the plasma membrane of the sarcoplasmic reticulum decreases $[Ca^{2+}]_i$ by inducing both a Ca^{2+} extrusion (outside the cell) and a Ca^{2+} sequestration (in the sarcoplasmic reticulum) (Fig. 5) [38]. Cyclic guanosine monophosphate kinase also reduces $[Ca^{2+}]_i$ by decreasing Ca^{2+} entry in the cell. This decreased entry seems to be due to the inhibition of L-type Ca^{2+} channels (a voltage-dependent Ca^{2+} channel) as a result of a direct effect of the kinase on the channel [38,39]. In addition, cGMP-kinase may open a plasmalemmal K^+ channel (e.g. the ATP-sensitive K^+ ($K_{(ATP)}$) channel) [40]. This opening induces a K^+ efflux which causes a loss of positive charges by the cell and leads to membrane hyperpolarization. This, in turn, closes the L-type Ca^{2+} channel. Finally, cGMP-kinase has been shown to cause an inhibition of the agonist-induced formation of the second messenger, inositol trisphosphate [38]. Since this messenger stimulates the mobilization of intracellular Ca^{2+} [41], cGMP-kinase may decrease $[Ca^{2+}]_i$ in this way.

The third mechanism for a cirrhosis-induced reduction in $[Ca^{2+}]_i$ bypasses cyclic nucleotide pathways [36]. This mechanism occurs with certain vasodilators such as PGI_2, neuropeptides (i.e. CGRP and VIP) and beta$_2$-adrenergic agonists. These agents may induce vasodilatation by a mechanism which bypasses cyclic nucleotide pathways [36]. Indeed, these substances are known to open $K_{(ATP)}$ channels *in vitro* and $K_{(ATP)}$ channel results in membrane hyperpolarization and vasorelaxation (see above and [42]). Evidence has been provided that $K_{(ATP)}$ channel opening was abnormally increased in aortic smooth-muscle cells from rats with cirrhosis [43].

Since all vasodilator mechanisms which are hyperstimulated in cirrhosis decrease vascular tone by decreasing $[Ca^{2+}]_i$ (see above), an inhibition of these mechanisms should increase $[Ca^{2+}]_i$ and reduce cirrhosis-induced vasodilatation. This goal could be reached by the inhibition of the cyclic nucleotide (cGMP or cAMP) synthesis or the blockade of $K_{(ATP)}$ channels (Fig. 5).

The inhibition of cGMP synthesis can be achieved by the reduction in NO synthesis. In fact, it has been shown that several inhibitors of NO synthesis increased the vascular resistance in systemic and splanchnic territories in portal hypertensive rats [44–47]. However, NO inhibition did not decrease portal pressure in these studies. Cyclic guanosine monophosphate synthesis can also be reduced by the inhibition of soluble guanylyl cyclase, for example by methylene blue. Thus, it has been shown that this substance increased systemic vascular resistance in patients with cirrhosis [48]. The inhibition of cAMP synthesis can be achieved by decreasing the production of substances

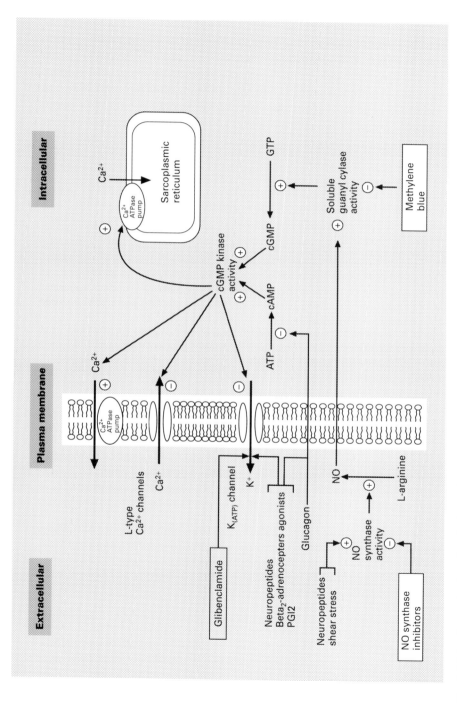

Fig. 5 Molecular mechanisms by which vasodilators decrease vascular tone. +, activation; −, inhibition.

which stimulate this synthesis. For example, a decrease in PGI_2 production as a result of inhibiting cyclooxygenase (with indomethacin) reduces cAMP synthesis [49]. Indomethacin has been shown to increase the vascular resistance in systemic and splanchnic territories in portal hypertensive rats [49,50]. Finally, the blockade of $K_{(ATP)}$ channels is obtained with sulphonylureas such as glibenclamide [51]. In fact, glibenclamide has been shown to increase in systemic and splanchnic vascular resistances in rats with portal hypertension [51,52]. Clinical studies are, however, needed which would be based on data provided by molecular pharmacological investigations.

REFERENCES

1 Brenner DA, Alcorn JM. Therapy for hepatic fibrosis. *Semin Liver Dis* 1990; **10**: 75–83.

2 Rojkind M. Fibrogenesis in cirrhosis. Potential for therapeutic intervention. *Pharmacol Ther* 1991; **53**: 81–104.

3 Lin HC, Soubrane O, Cailmail S, Lebrec D. Early chronic administration of propranolol reduces the severity of portal hypertension and portal-systemic shunts in conscious portal vein stenosed rats. *J Hepatol* 1991; **13**: 213–219.

4 Lin HC, Soubrane O, Lebrec D. Prevention of portal hypertension and portosystemic shunts by early chronic administration of clonidine in conscious portal vein-stenosed rats. *Hepatology* 1991; **14**: 325–330.

5 Sarin SK, Groszmann RJ, Mosca PG *et al*. Propranolol ameliorates the development of portal-systemic shunting in a chronic murine schistosomiasis model of portal hypertension. *J Clin Invest* 1991; **87**: 1032–1036.

6 Hayes PC, Crichton S, Shepherd AN, Bouchier IAD. Propranolol in chronic liver disease: a controlled trial of its effect and safety over twelve months. *Q J Med* 1987; **246**: 823–834.

7 Plevris JN, Elliot R, Mills PR *et al*. Effect of propranolol on prevention of first variceal bleed and survival in patients with chronic liver disease. *Aliment Pharmacol Ther* 1994; **8**: 63–70.

8 Lebrec D. Pharmacological treatment of portal hypertension: hemodynamic effects and prevention of bleeding. *Pharmacol Ther* 1994; **62**: 65–107.

9 Mills PR, Rae AP, Farah DA, Russell RI, Lorimer AR, Carter DC. Comparison of three adrenoreceptor blocking agents in patients with cirrhosis and portal hypertension. *Gut* 1984; **26**: 73–78.

10 Albillos A, Banares R, Barrios C *et al*. Oral administration of clonidine in patients with alcoholic cirrhosis. Hemodynamic and liver function effects. *Gastroenterology* 1992; **102**: 248–254.

11 Roulot D, Moreau R, Gaudin C *et al*. Long-term sympathetic and hemodynamic responses to clonidine in patients with cirrhosis and ascites. *Gastroenterology* 1992; **102**, 1309–1318.

12 Klein CP. Spironolacton in der Behandlung der portalen Hypertonic bei Leberzirrhose. *Dtsch Med Wochenschr* 1985; **110**: 1774–1776.

13 Okumura H, Aramaki T, Katsuta Y *et al*. Reduction in hepatic venous pressure gradient as a consequence of volume contraction due to chronic administration of spironolactone in patients with cirrhosis and no ascites. *Am J Gastroenterol* 1991; **86**: 46–52.

14 Garcia-Pagan JC, Salmeron JM, Feu F *et al*. Effects of low-sodium diet and spir-
    onolactone on portal pressure in patients with compensated cirrhosis. *Hepatology*
    1994; **19**: 1095–1099.

15 Huet PM, Pomier-Layrargues G, Semret M. Effects of ritanserin, a serotonin antagonist
    in cirrhotic patients with portal hypertension. *Hepatology* 1988; **8**: 1422.

16 Vorobioff J, Garcia-Tsao G, Groszmann R *et al*. Long-term hemodynamic effects of
    Ketanserin, a 5-hydroxytryptamine blocker, in portal hypertensive patients. *J. Hepatol*
    1989; **8**: 88–91.

17 Garcia-Pagan J, Feu F, Navasa S *et al*. Long-term haemodynamic effects of isosorbide
    5-mononitrate in patients with cirrhosis and portal hypertension. *J Hepatol* 1990; **11**:
    189–195.

18 Cervinka J, Kordac V, Kalab M. Effect of per oral administration of isosorbide dini-
    trate on portal pressure and blood flow in patients with cirrhosis of the liver. *J Int Med
    Res* 1989; **17**: 560–564.

19 Freeman JG, Barton JR, Record CO. Effect of isosorbide dinitrate, verapammil and
    labetalol on portal pressure in cirrhosis. *Br Med J* 1985; **291**: 561–562.

20 Vorobioff J, Picabea E, Gamen M, Villavicencio R. Isosorbide dinitrate in portal
    hypertensive patients. *J Hepatol* 1992; **16**: 387.

21 Hüppe D, Jéger D, Tromm A, Tunn S, Barmeyer J, May B. Acute and long-term effects
    of molsidomine on portal and cardiac haemodynamics in patients with cirrhosis of the
    liver. *Eur J Gastroenterol Hepatol* 1992; **4**: 849–855.

22 Angelico M, Carli L, Piat C *et al*. Isosorbide-5-mononitrate vs propranolol in the
    prevention of first bleeding in cirrhosis. *Gastroenterology* 1993; **104**: 1460–1465.

23 Garcia-Pagan JC, Navasa M, Bosch J, Bru C, Pizcueta P, Rodés J. Enhancement of
    portal pressure reduction by the association of isosorbide-5-mononitrate to propra-
    nolol administration in patients with cirrhosis. *Hepatology* 1990; **11**: 230–238.

24 Monnin JL, Vinal JP, Le Quellec A *et al*. Etude par échographie Doppler pulsé des effets
    de la molsidomine et de l'association propranolol–molsidomine sur l'hémodynamique
    portale. *Gastroenterol Clin Biol* 1992; **16**: 745–750.

25 Morillas RM, Planas RR, Cabré E *et al*. Propranolol plus isosorbide-5- mononitrate for
    portal hypertension in cirrhosis: long-term hemodynamic and renal effects. *Hepatology*
    1994; **20** 1502–1508.

26 Aramaki T, Sekiyama T, Katsuta Y *et al*. Long-term hemodynamic effects of a 4-week
    regimen of nipradilol, a new β-blocker with nitrovasodilating properties, in patients
    with portal hypertension due to cirrhosis. A comparative study with propranolol. *J
    Hepatol* 1992; **15**: 48–53.

27 Hadengue A, Lee SS, Moreau R, Braillon A, Lebrec D. Beneficial hemodynamic effects
    of ketanserin in patients with cirrhosis: possible role of serotonergic mechanisms in
    portal hypertension. *Hepatology* 1987; **7**: 644–647.

28 Pomier-Layrargues G, Giroux L, Rocheleau B, Huet PM. Combined treatment of
    portal hypertension with ritanserin and propranolol in conscious and unrestrained
    cirrhotic rats. *Hepatology* 1992; **15**: 878–882.

29 Roulot D, Gaudin C, Braillon A, Sekiyama T, Bacq Y, Lebrec D. Hemodynamic effects
    of combination of clonidine and propranolol in conscious cirrhotic rats. *Can J Physiol
    Pharmacol* 1989; **67**: 1369–1372.

30 Garcia-Pagan JC, Salmeron JM, Feu F *et al*. Spironolactone (Sp) decreases portal
    pressure in patients with compensated cirrhosis. *J Hepatol* 1992; **13** (Suppl. 2): S30.

31 Sogni P, Soupison T, Moreau R *et al*. Hemodynamic effects of acute administration of
    furosemide in patients with cirrhosis receiving β-adrenergic antagonists. *J Hepatol*

1994; **20**: 548–552.

32 Sharma NR, Davis MJ. Mechanism of substance P-induced hyperpolarization of porcine coronary artery endothelial cells. *Am J Physiol* 1994; **266**: H256–H164.

33 Murthy KS, Makhlouf GM. Vasoactive intestinal peptide/pituitary adenylate cyclase-activating peptide-dependent activation of membrane-bound NO synthase in smooth muscle mediated by pertussis toxin-sensitive G_{i1-2}*. *J Biol Chem* 1994; **269**: 15977–15980.

34 Gray DW, Marshall I. Human α-calcitonin gene-related peptide stimulates adenylate cyclase and guanylate cyclase and relaxes rat thoracic aorta by releasing nitric oxide. *Br J Pharmacol* 1992; **107**: 691–696.

35 Moncada S, Palmer RMJ, Higgs EA. Nitric oxide: physiology, pathophysiology, and pharmacology. *Pharmacol Rev* 1991; **43**: 109–142.

36 Moreau R, Lebrec D. Endogenous factors involved in the control of arterial tone in cirrhosis. *J Hepatol* 1995; **22**: 370–376.

37 Rembold CM. Regulation of contraction and relaxation in arterial smooth muscle. *Hypertension* 1992; **20**: 129–137.

38 Lincoln TM, Cornwell TL. Intracellular cyclic GMP receptor proteins. *FASEB J* 1993; **7**: 328–338.

39 Meriney SD, Gray DB, Pilar GR. Somatostatin-induced inhibition of neuronal Ca^{2+} current modulated by cGMP-dependent protein kinase. *Nature* 1994; **369**: 336–339.

40 Kubo M, Nakaya Y, Matsuoka S, Saito K, Kuroda Y. Atrial natriuretic factor and isosorbide dinitrate modulate the gating of ATP-sensitive K^+ channels in cultured vascular smooth muscle cells. *Circ Res* 1994; **74**: 471–476.

41 Berridge MJ. Inositol trisphosphate and calcium signalling. *Nature* 1993; **361**: 315–325.

42 Standen NB, Quayle JM, Davies NW, Brayden JE, Huang Y, Nelson MT. Hyperpolarizing vasodilators activate ATP-sensitive K^+ channels in arterial smooth muscle. *Science* 1989; **245**: 177–180.

43 Moreau R, Rona JP, Cornel D *et al.* Metabolic inhibition results in an abnormal increase in outward K^+ currents in arterial smooth muscle cells of rats with cirrhosis. *Hepatology* 1994; **20**: 98A.

44 Piczueta MP, Pique JM, Bosch J, Whittle BRJ, Moncada S. Effects of inhibiting nitric oxide biosynthesis on the systemic and splanchnic circulation of rats with portal hypertension. *Br J Pharmacol* 1992; **105**: 184–190.

45 Lee FY, Albillos A, Colombato LA, Groszmann R. The role of nitric oxide in the vascular hyporesponsiveness to methoxamine in portal hypertensive rats. *Hepatology* 1992; **16**: 1043–1048.

46 Iwata F, Joh T, Kawai T, Itoh M. Role of EDRF in splanchnic blood flow of normal and chronic portal hypertensive rats. *Am J Physiol* 1992; **263**: G149–G154.

47 Pilette C, Kistetter P, Sogni P, Cailmail S, Moreau R, Lebrec D. The effects of a nitric oxide biosynthesis inhibitor on hyperdynamic circulation in two models of portal hypertensive rats. *J Hepatol Gastroenterol* 1995 (in press).

48 Midgley S, Grant IS, Haynes WG, Webb DJ. Nitric oxide in liver failure. *Lancet* 1991; **338**: 1590.

49 Oberti F, Sogni P, Cailmail S, Moreau R, Pipy B, Lebrec D. Role of prostacyclin in hemodynamic alterations in conscious rats with extra- or intra-hepatic portal hypertension. *Hepatology* 1993; **18**: 621–627.

50 Wu Y, Burns RC, Sitzman JV. Effects of nitric oxide and cyclooxygenase inhibition on splanchnic hemodynamics in portal hypertension. *Hepatology* 1993; **18**: 1416–1421.

51 Moreau R, Komeichi H, Kirstetter P, Ohsuga M, Cailmail S, Lebrec D. Altered control of vascular tone by adenosine triphosphate-sensitive potassium channels in rats with cirrhosis. *Gastroenterology* 1994; **106**: 1016–1023.

52 Moreau R, Komeichi H, Cailmail S, Lebrec D. Blockade of ATP-sensitive K$^+$ channels by glibenclamide reduces portal pressure and hyperkinetic circulation in portal hypertensive rats. *J Hepatol* 1992; **16**: 215–218.

Recent Advances in the Endoscopic Management of Variceal Bleeding

Simon G.J. Williams and David Westaby

INTRODUCTION

Variceal haemorrhage may occur in up to 30% of patients with chronic liver disease [1], with an estimated mortality of 50% for the initial bleed [2] and a 30% in-hospital mortality for subsequent bleeds.

Endoscopic techniques have been used to treat variceal haemorrhage for over 50 years [3]. They are now accepted as the first-line treatment for active variceal bleeding [4,5] as well as for the prevention of recurrent haemorrhage [5,6]. While injection sclerotherapy controls active haemorrhage in approximately 90% of cases [7,8], rebleeding occurs in up to 55% [9] and it is of questionable benefit for cardia/fundal gastric varices [10]. In the absence of a safe and effective alternative treatment, sclerotherapy complication rates of up to 40%, which are largely the result of sclerosant-induced mucosal damage, and mortality rates of up to 2% have been accepted [11,12].

In the light of these limitations the search for improvements in the application of injection sclerotherapy and for alternative endoscopic treatments for the management of variceal haemorrhage continues.

INJECTION SCLEROTHERAPY

It is well recognized that the number of sessions required to achieve variceal obliteration has varied both within and between series. It has been hypothesized that these differences can be attributed to the variation in the venous anatomy in the distal oesophagus, and in particular to the presence of perforating veins communicating between the intrinsic and paraoesophageal vessels. These perforating veins have been confirmed both by *in vivo* Doppler ultrasound [13] and from post-mortem studies [14].

A recent study has confirmed the importance of these perforating vessels in the clinical setting by demonstrating the need for a prolonged series of sclerotherapy sessions in those in whom perforating vessels had been demonstrated. Using computed tomography, these investigators were able to show that patients with paraoesophageal varices required more treatment sessions, more sclerosant and longer periods of time to achieve variceal obliteration [15]. In addition, varices reappeared at an earlier stage in more of those patients in whom oesophageal perforating vessels had been demonstrated. The most distal perforating vessels reliably occur 3–5 cm above the gastro-oesophageal junction and as such sclerotherapy should extend up to 5 cm proximal to the gastro-oesophageal junction.

COMBINATION OF INJECTION SCLEROTHERAPY WITH PHARMACOLOGICAL AGENTS

Pharmacological agents have been widely investigated and applied for the control of variceal haemorrhage. More recently attention has focused on the addition of pharmacological agents to injection sclerotherapy either in the acute setting or the immediate period following the acute application of sclerotherapy in an attempt to improve efficacy.

Agents aimed at reducing splanchnic inflow

Propranolol

A number of trials have combined oral propranol and injection sclerotherapy. The results of these trials are conflicting, perhaps reflecting the small numbers of patients recruited [16,17].

Isosorbide-5-mononitrate

It has been clearly demonstrated that nitrates reduce splanchnic inflow [18] and might, therefore, be expected to reduce rebleeding after injection sclerotherapy.

A recently reported study suggests that the use of isosorbide-5-mononitrate, in a slow-release preparation at a dose of 50 mg/day, and prescribed following the index session of sclerotherapy, has the effect of reducing rebleeding up to the time of variceal eradication (with 10.8% of patients on active treatment compared with 38.4% of patients on placebo having a rebleed) [19]. However, the benefits with regard to rebleeding may be offset by a significant (20%) reduction in glomerular filtration rate [20] which may result in problems with the management of ascites [21].

Somatostatin/octreotide

There has been increasing attention devoted to somatostatin and its long-acting analogue, octreotide, in the control of acute variceal haemorrhage. A continuous infusion of somatostatin controls bleeding in 40–77% of cases [22], and there are reports of similar efficacy for octreotide [23,24]. These agents have the advantage of very few side effects. Additional interest in somatostatin has followed evidence that an infusion, started before sclerotherapy and continued over the 5 days following the index bleed, is associated with a reduction in rebleeding rates [25,26].

Agents directed at reducing or ameliorating mucosal damage

Mucosal ulceration following injection sclerotherapy has been identified as the source of rebleeding in up to 20% of patients [27]. This ulceration may be more extensive and protracted in patients with advanced liver disease [28]. Attention has, therefore, focused on drugs which may alter the natural history of bleeding from such mucosal damage.

Sucralfate

A large controlled trial has confirmed the efficacy of the mucosal protectant sucralfate in the reduction of early rebleeding and of rebleeding up to the time of variceal obliteration [27]. The benefits observed in this study occurred without evidence of more rapid ulcer healing suggesting that sucralfate may exhibit a direct haemostatic effect.

Omeprazole

The proton pump inhibitor omeprazole is highly effective at healing both acute and chronic postsclerotherapy ulcers [29,30]. This suggests that chronic ulcers, which may be the source of both pain and rebleeding, may be maintained by acid pepsin.

ALTERNATIVES TO INJECTION SCLEROTHERAPY

Endoscopic banding ligation

Banding ligation was first reported in humans in 1990 [31], and represents an important development in the endoscopic treatment of varices. The technique uses the same concepts as those applied to banding ligation of internal haemorrhoids. Following the initial diagnostic endoscopy, an overtube is passed over the endoscope into the oesophagus to allow repeated intubation of the oesophagus. A cylinder is then attached to the end of a forward-viewing endoscope and a second cylinder is inserted into this. A prestressed rubber band is positioned at the distal end of the inner cylinder which is held in place by a 'trip' wire running through the biopsy channel of the endoscope. The device is closely apposed to the variceal cord, suction is applied through the endoscope, and the band is released over the entrapped varix by pulling the trip wire. Application of the bands is commenced at the gastro-oesophageal junction and then worked proximally in a helical fashion for approximately 5 cm until six to eight bands have been applied. The entrapped varix sloughs off leaving a small discrete ulcer.

There are currently three major trials reporting controlled comparison of injection sclerotherapy with banding ligation [32–34]. The results of these three studies comparing acute and long-term banding ligation and sclerotherapy are broadly similar. For active bleeding all three trials showed no specific advantage for either treatment. Banding ligation controlled bleeding in 82–89% of cases identified as actively bleeding at the time of the index endoscopy as compared with 77–89% for those treated by injection sclerotherapy.

Comparison of the long-term results revealed some variation between the three trials, and it should be noted that one of the studies randomized a significantly higher number of patients with high Child–Pugh scores to the banding ligation group (34 vs. 13%), making interpretation of these data more difficult [34].

Only one study reported a statistically significant reduction in rebleeding in the banding cohort (30 vs. 53%) [33] while there was a trend towards less frequent rebleeding in the other two trials (36 vs. 48% [32] and 24 vs. 31% [34]). The reduction in bleeding may be attributable to more rapid variceal obliteration (see below) with banding ligation, or alternatively to the fact that banding ligation tends to result in larger, but shallower, ulcers than sclerotherapy [35]. This study of oesophageal ulceration induced by the two techniques showed that the ulcers produced by variceal ligation were, on average, 0.6 mm deep with a mean surface area of 85.4 mm^2 as compared with ulcers of 1.8 mm depth and 13.3 mm^2 surface area produced by injection sclerotherapy [35].

With regard to the efficacy of banding ligation as long-term therapy for oesophageal varices there was a statistically significant reduction in the number of sessions required to achieve variceal obliteration in two of the trials (3.4 vs. 4.9 sessions; 39 vs. 72 days [33], 4.1 vs. 6.2 sessions [34]), with a trend towards statistical significance in the other study (4 vs. 5 [32]).

Reported complications of banding ligation were very few (see Table 14). Two of the studies report a statistically significant reduction in complications in the banding ligation group (2 vs. 22% [32] and 24 vs. 56% [34]), although much of the difference is attributable to the high frequency (12 and 33%, respectively) of oesophageal strictures in the sclerotherapy group. A stricture

Table 14 Complications of banding ligation.

Oesophageal ulceration
Rebleeding from oesophageal ulceration
Oesophageal trauma associated with overtube insertion
Bacteraemia
Bacterial peritonitis
Pneumonia

rate of 33% is much higher than previously reported and may, in this study, be related to the relatively high concentration of the sclerosing agent (3% sodium tetradecylsulphate mixed 1 : 1 with 50% dextrose) and relatively large volumes of sclerosant injected (mean of 9.3 ml).

Mortality data are incomplete due to relatively short follow-up (median < 1 year), but one of the American studies does report improved survival in the banding ligation group (18 vs. 45%) [35]. The authors attribute the improved survival to reduced complications associated with banding ligation.

One further study has compared the use of injection sclerotherapy and banding ligation for acute bleeding, with all patients being subsequently treated by injection sclerotherapy [36]. This study examines whether or not banding ligation at the index endoscopy will result in earlier and more successful control of bleeding varices in the long term. Banding ligation resulted in fewer complications in the short term and the need for significantly less sclerosant to achieve variceal obliteration thereafter (23.9 vs. 39.0 ml; $P < 0.0001$). This reduction in volume of sclerosant might presumably result in fewer sclerotherapy-related complications in the long term and perhaps reflects the effectiveness of banding ligation in achieving a rapid reduction in varix size. However, if the treatment reduces variceal size more quickly and is associated with fewer treatment-related complications it would seem logical to apply banding ligation in the long term to achieve variceal obliteration.

Thus, these initial studies suggest that endoscopic banding ligation is a promising technique for the treatment of oesophageal varices, with the potential for faster variceal obliteration, fewer treatment-related complications, and possibly less rebleeding and a reduction in mortality.

However, several caveats remain. While the technique is simple it is relatively cumbersome, with a session of banding ligation taking up to 30 minutes [37], and potential difficulties placing the 27-cm long overtube. Furthermore, the field of vision is reduced by about 30% with the banding device attached. These limitations are particularly problematic in the acute setting where a prolonged procedure in a sick patient is undesirable and where effective placement of the rubber bands may be hampered by the reduced field of vision coupled with large volumes of fresh blood refluxing up the oesophagus. It may be more appropriate, therefore, to use injection sclerotherapy to control haemorrhage in the patient who is actively bleeding at the index endoscopy and to reserve banding ligation for the patient who has clearly bled but who has stopped bleeding spontaneously.

GASTRIC VARICES

Gastric varices may be the source of haemorrhage in up to 36% of patients presenting with bleeding varices [10]. The strategies available for the treatment of gastric varices are different from those applied to bleeding oesophageal varices. While injection sclerotherapy has been applied to treat active bleeding from gastric varices, it has been demonstrated that its use in cardia/fundal varices is associated with a high rate of rebleeding and a frequent need to resort to surgical intervention [38].

While there is speculation that banding ligation may be more effective in the control of bleeding from such isolated fundal gastric varices, with limited reports in the literature [39], there are now two alternative injectates which appear to be effective in controlling fundal variceal haemorrhage and which may also be applied to varices located elsewhere in the upper gastrointestinal tract.

The tissue adhesives

The tissue adhesives *n*-butyl-2-cyanoacrylate (Histoacryl) and isobutyl-2-cyanoacrylate (Bucrylate) have been used to treat both oesophageal and gastric varices [40,41], although the latter agent has been removed from the European market because of concerns about carcinogenicity [42]. Control of bleeding has been reported in about 90% of cases. The adhesives harden within seconds of coming into contact with blood, and within a few minutes when activated by water [43]. Thus, their injection, if executed correctly, should result in almost immediate control of bleeding as the lumen of the varix is occluded. However, the rapid hardening of the adhesives means that their application is not as simple as that of conventional sclerosants. The technique requires care to ensure that the adhesive does not come into contact with the endoscope and thus result in permanent damage to the channels of the instrument. This risk can be minimized by applying silicone oil to the tip of the instrument and by mixing the adhesive with a radiographic contrast agent (Lipiodol), in a ratio of 1:1, to delay premature hardening [40]. This modification allows the localization of the injected adhesive on a radiograph and may allow the monitoring of injections, although the clinical importance of such an approach is unclear [44]. A further modification of the technique is to ensure that the needle is correctly placed within the varix by employing a trial injection of distilled water. Once correct placement has been confirmed, the tissue adhesive is injected in 0.5–1.0 ml aliquots. Should the adhesive leak, the endoscope can be withdrawn and cleaned before the polymer has a chance to set.

The histological changes in autopsy specimens obtained soon after adhesive injection show diffusion of polymer into the wall of the viscus in association with mucosal ulceration [45]. Several weeks later (2 weeks to 3 months) the overlying mucosa sloughs off and a glue cast is extruded into the lumen of the gastrointestinal tract [46]. The ulceration subsequently re-epithelializes.

While reports of the use of these agents in the control of active gastric variceal haemorrhage are rather limited, there is one large report of the uncontrolled use of Bucrylate in 27 patients bleeding from gastric varices [41]. The majority of patients were Child–Pugh grade A or B, and seven were actively bleeding at the time of the index endoscopy. Active bleeding was stopped in six patients, none of whom was bleeding heavily, thus allowing adequate views of the gastric fundus to be obtained. Two of these patients rebled within 6 hours and responded to a further injection of tissue adhesive, while the seventh stopped bleeding spontaneously and was injected at a second endoscopy. There were 16 episodes of rebleeding, one of these being attributable to mucosal ulceration and one from a varix that was ejecting an adhesive cast, four from gastric varices alone which responded to further injections of tissue adhesive and four in a single patient who was bleeding from oesophagogastric varices and who failed to respond to further injections of Bucrylate. Variceal obliteration was achieved in 70% of patients with one to two sessions of Bucrylate injection of one to eight injections each. There were eight deaths over a mean follow-up of 14.7 months, but none of these was attributable to gastric variceal bleeding.

The results of this study are encouraging when compared with the use of conventional sclerosants to control gastric variceal haemorrhage [47]. Conventional sclerosants are associated with mucosal ulceration that delays variceal eradication and frequently leads to rebleeding and perforation. Rebleeding from postinjection variceal ulceration is a major complication of injection sclerotherapy [48] but, on the basis of this report, does not seem to be as common and is apparently easier to control with the tissue adhesives [41].

A number of worrying complications have been attributed to the tissue adhesives. In one series, three deaths were attributed directly to mediastinitis caused by the adhesive [49] and of even greater concern are two reported cerebrovascular accidents attributable directly to dissemination of the tissue adhesive into the cerebral circulation [50].

Thrombin

The use of human and bovine thrombin as a constituent of a thrombogenic cocktail has been widely reported [51–53]. Initial concerns about distant and disseminated thrombosis have not been confirmed, although some derangement of the clotting cascade can be detected upon detailed analysis [54].

Thrombin injection does not require the technical precautions necessary for the tissue adhesives and is performed using the freehand injection technique used for injection sclerotherapy.

In uncontrolled series thrombin appears to be effective in controlling haemorrhage from both oesophageal and gastric varices [53]. One series concentrates on its uncontrolled use for the treatment of gastric varices in 11 consecutive patients [55].

Seven of the patients were Child–Pugh grade A and B, and nine were deemed to have bled from fundal/greater curve gastric varices. Four were actively bleeding at the index endoscopy (three from the fundus), although in one of these patients adequate views were not obtained of the gastric fundus due to a large amount of adherent clot and it was only at the subsequent endoscopy that this was confirmed as the source of the bleed. Patients were injected intravariceally with bovine thrombin (Armour Pharmaceutical Co., Illinois, USA) reconstituted to 1000 units/ml. Haemostasis for the presenting episode was achieved in all patients with a single session of thrombin injection. A median of two injections was required to achieve variceal obliteration. A mean volume of 5.5 ml of thrombin was used at each injection session. Patients were followed-up for up to 13 months.

The only complication reported in this series was of rebleeding, which occurred in three patients, but originated from gastric varices in only one. In the context of the experience with both conventional sclerosants and the tissue adhesives, the absence of any evidence of mucosal ulceration and consequently rebleeding attributable to this is clearly important. Also of importance was the absence of any evidence of allergic/anaphylactic reactions to bovine thrombin, despite repeated treatments, or of thrombosis distant from the site of injection [53,55].

This initial experience with gastric varices suggests that thrombin is an important addition to the endoscopist's options in the treatment of bleeding fundal gastric varices. It is important to note, however, that the series was small and uncontrolled.

SUMMARY

While injection sclerotherapy is effective in the control of oesophageal variceal haemorrhage, it has well-documented limitations and complications.

The addition of pharmacological agents may improve efficacy, as in the demonstration that the injection of sclerosant at the level of the perforating vessels 3–5 cm proximal to the oesophagogastric junction is important in achieving control of haemorrhage and earlier variceal eradication.

The advent of endoscopic banding ligation is perhaps the most significant advance, with a clear demonstration of equal efficacy to injection sclerotherapy in the control of haemorrhage and perhaps an important reduction in complications. However, long-term data are still awaited. For the first time the endoscopist has more than one option for the management of gastro-oesophageal varices.

It is now feasible to select the appropriate therapy on the basis of the clinical setting. Acute injection sclerotherapy remains a quick and simple technique for the control of active bleeding from oesophageal varices, and could be followed 2 or 3 days later by banding ligation. Earlier obliteration of varices with this technique may offer the prospect of only two or three sessions of therapy. The availability of the tissue adhesives and thrombin as injectates for fundal gastric varices provide the option of an initial attempt at endoscopic therapy in this high-risk group.

REFERENCES

1 Cales P, Pascal JP. Histoire naturelle des varices oesophagiennes au cours de la cirrhose (de la naissance à la rupture). *Gastroenterol Clin Biol* 1988; **12**: 245–254.

2 Christensen E, Fauerholdt L, Schlichting P *et al.* Aspects of the natural history of gastrointestinal bleeding in cirrhosis and the effect of prednisolone. *Gastroenterology* 1981; **81**: 944–952.

3 Crafoord C, Freckner P. New surgical treatment of varicose veins of the oesophagus. *Acta Otolaryngol (Stockholm)* 1939; **27**: 422–429.

4 Paquet K-J, Feussner H. Endoscopic sclerosis and esophageal balloon tamponade in acute haemorrhage from esophago-gastric varices: a prospective controlled randomized trial. *Hepatology* 1985; **5**: 580–583.

5 Westaby D, MacDougall BRD, Williams R. Improved survival following injection sclerotherapy for oesophageal varices: final analysis of a controlled trial. *Hepatology* 1985; **5**: 627–631.

6 Barsoum MS, Boulous FI, El-Rooby A, Risk-Allah MA, Ibrahim AS. Tamponade and injection sclerotherapy in the management of bleeding oesopageal varices. *Br J Surg* 1982; **69**: 76–78.

7 Prindiville T, Trudeau W. A comparison of immediate versus delayed endoscopic injection sclerosis of bleeding oesophageal varices. *Gastrointest Endosc* 1986; **32**: 385–388.

8 Westaby D, Hayes P, Gimson AE, Polson RJ, Williams R. Controlled trial of injection sclerotherapy for active variceal bleeding. *Hepatology* 1989; **9**: 274–277.

9 MacDougall BRD, Westaby D, Theodossi A, Dawson JL, Williams R. Increased long-term survival in variceal haemorrhage using injection sclerotherapy. Results of a controlled trial. *Lancet* 1982; **i**: 124–127.

10 Merican I, Burroughs AK. Gastric varices. *Eur J Gastroenterol Hepatol* 1991; **4**: 511–520.

11 Schuman BM, Beckman, JW, Tedesco FJ, Griffin JW, Assad R. Complications of injection sclerotherapy: a review. *Am J Gastroenterol* 1987; **82**: 823–829.

12 Infante-Rivard C, Esnaola S, Villneuve JR. Role of endoscopic sclerotherapy in long-term management of variceal bleeding: a meta-analysis. *Gastroenterology* 1989; **96**: 1087–1092.

13 MacCormack TT, Rose JD, Smith PM, Johnson AG. Perforating veins and blood flow in oesophageal varices. *Lancet* 1983; **ii**: 1442–1444.

14 Vianna A, Hayes PC, Moscosco G *et al*. Normal venous circulation of the gastro-esophageal junction: a route to understanding varices. *Gastroenterology* 1987; **93**: 876–889.

15 Lin CY, Lin PW, Tsai HM, Lin XZ, Chang TT, Shin JS. Influence of paraesophageal venous collaterals on efficacy of endoscopic sclerotherapy for esophageal varices. *Hepatology* 1994; **19**: 602–608.

16 Hayes PC. Prevention of recurrent variceal bleeding: pharmacologic measures. In: Westaby D (ed.), *Variceal Bleeding. Gastrointestinal Endoscopy Clinics of North America*. Philadelphia: W.B. Saunders, 1992: 137–150.

17 Blei AT. Portal hypertension. *Current Opin Gastroenterol* 1994; **10**: 295–302.

18 Alvarez D, Mastai R, Lennie A, Soifer G, Levi D, Terg R. Non-invasive measurement of portal venous blood flow in patients with cirrhosis: effects of physiological and pharmacological stimuli. *Dig Dis Sci* 1991; **36**: 82–86.

19 Bertoni G, Sassatelli R, Fornaciari G *et al*. Oral isosorbide-5-mononitrate reduces the rebleeding rate during the course of injection sclerotherapy for esophageal varices. *Scand J Gastroenterol* 1994; **29**: 363–370.

20 Salmeron JM, Ruiz del Arbol L, Gines A *et al*. Renal effects of acute isosorbide-5-mononitrate administration in cirrhosis. *Hepatology* 1993; **17**: 800–806.

21 Vorobioff J, Picabea E, Gamen M *et al*. Propranolol compared with propranolol plus isosorbide dinitrate in portal-hypertensive patients: long-term haemodynamic and renal effects. *Hepatology* 1993; **18**: 477–484.

22 Burroughs AK. Medical management of bleeding oesophageal varices. *Dig Dis* 1992; **10** (Suppl. 1): 30–37.

23 McKee R. A study of octreotide in oesophageal varices. *Digestion* 1990; **45** (Suppl. 1): 60–65.

24 Sung JJY, Chung SCS, Lai C-W *et al*. Octreotide infusion or emergency sclerotherapy for variceal haemorrhage. *Lancet* 1993; **I**: 637–641.

25 Shields R, Jenkins SA, Baxter JN *et al*. A prospective randomised controlled trial comparing the efficacy of somatostatin with injection sclerotherapy in the control of bleeding oesophageal varices. *J Hepatol* 1992; **16**: 128–137.

26 Burroughs AK. Somatostatin and octreotide for variceal bleeding. *J Hepatol* 1991; **13**: 1–4.

27 Polson RJ, Westaby D, Gimson AES *et al*. Sucralfate for the prevention of early rebleeding following injection sclerotherapy for oesophageal varices. *Hepatology* 1989; **10**: 279–282.

28 Singhal A, Sarin SK, Sood GK, Broor SL. Ulcers after intravariceal sclerotherapy – correlation of symptoms and factors affecting healing. *J Clin Gastroenterol* 1990; **12**: 250–254.

29 Shepherd H, Barkin JS. Omeprazole heals mucosal ulcers associated with endoscopic injection sclerotherapy. *Gastrointest Endosc* 1991; **39**: 474–475.

30 Gimson A, Polson R, Westaby D, Williams R. Omeprazole in the management of intractable oesophageal ulceration following injection sclerotherapy. *Gastroenterology* 1990; **99**: 1829–1831.

31 Stiegmann GV, Goff JS, Sun JH, Hruza D, Reveille RM. Endoscopic ligation of esophageal varices. *Am J Surg* 1990; **159**: 21–62.

32 Stiegmann GV, Goff JS, Michaletz-Onody PA *et al*. Endoscopic sclerotherapy as compared with endoscopic ligation for bleeding esophageal varices. *N Engl J Med* 1992; **326**: 1527–1532.

33 Gimson AES, Ramage JK, Panos MZ *et al*. Randomised trial of variceal banding ligation versus injection sclerotherapy for bleeding oesophageal varices. *Lancet* 1993; i: 391–394.

34 Laine L, El-Newihi HM, Migikovsky B, Sloane R, Garcia F. Endoscopic ligation compared with sclerotherapy for the treatment of bleeding esophageal varices. *Ann Intern Med* 1993; **119**: 1–7.

35 Young MF, Sanowski RA, Rasche R. Comparison and characterization of ulcerations induced by endoscopic ligation of esophageal varices versus endoscopic sclerotherapy. *Gastrointest Endosc* 1993; **39**: 119–122.

36 Hashizume M, Ohta M, Ueno K, Tanoue K, Kitano S, Sugimachi K. Endoscopic ligation of esophageal varices compared with injection sclerotherapy: a prospective randomized trial. *Gastrointest Endosc* 1993; **39**: 123–126.

37 Stiegmann GV, Cambre T, Sun JH. A new endoscopic elastic band ligating device. *Gastrointest Endosc* 1986; **32**: 230–233.

38 Gimson AES, Westaby D, Williams R. Endoscopic sclerotherapy in the management of gastric variceal haemorrhage. *J Hepatol* 1991; **13**: 274–278.

39 Sarin SK, Bhatia V. To ligate or sclerose: beginning of a new era in the management of esophageal varices? *Hepatology* 1993; **17**: 746–748.

40 Soehendra N, Grimm H, Nam V, Herger. N-Butyl-2-cyanoacrylate: a supplement to endoscopic sclerotherapy. *Endoscopy* 1987; **19**: 221–224.

41 Ramond M-J, Valla D, Mosnier J-F *et al*. Successful endoscopic obturation of gastric varices with butyl cyanoacrylate. *Hepatology* 1989; **10**: 488–493.

42 Gotlib J. Endoscopic obturation of esophageal and gastric varices with cyanoacrylic tissue adhesive. *Can J Gastroenterol* 1990; **4**: 637–638.

43 Yamamato M, Suzuki H. Endoscopic sclerotherapy with Histoacryl. *Dig Endosc* 1989; **6**: 851–857.

44 Stiegmann GV, Yamamato M. Endoscopic techniques for the management of active variceal bleeding. In: Westaby D (ed.), *Variceal Bleeding. Gastrointestinal Endoscopy Clinics of North America*. Philadelphia: WB Saunders, 1992: 59–75.

45 Fabiani B, Degott C, Ramond MJ *et al*. Obturation endoscopique des varices oeso-gastriques par le Bucrylate. *Gastroenterol Clin Biol* 1986; **10**: 580–583.

46 Yamamoto M, Otomi M, Suzuki H. Endoscopic injection sclerotherapy using Histoacryl. *Nippon Rinsho* 1990; **48**: 741–744.

47 Sarin SK, Lahoti D. Management of gastric varices. *Baillière Clin Gastroenterol* 1992; **6**: 527–548.

48 The Copenhagen Esophageal Varices Sclerotherapy Project. Sclerotherapy after first variceal haemorrhage in cirrhosis. A randomized multicenter trial. *N Engl J Med* 1984; **311**: 1594–1600.

49 Ramond MJ, Valla D, Gotlib JP, Rueff B, Benhamou JP. Obturation endoscopique des varices oeso-gastriques par le Bucrylate. *Gastroenterol Clin Biol* 1986; **10**: 575–579.

50 See A, Florent C, Lamy P, Levy VG, Bouvry M. Accidents vasculaires cerebaux apres obturation endoscopique des varices oesophagiennes par l'Isobutyl-2-cyanoacrylate chez deux malades. *Gastroenterol Clin Biol* 1986; **10**: 604–607.

51 Lyons SD, Sugawa C, Geller ER, Vandenberg DM. Comparison of 1% sodium tetradecyl sulphate to a thrombogenic sclerosant cocktail for endoscopic sclerotherapy. *Am Surg* 1988; **54**: 81–84.

52 Kitano S, Hashizume M, Yamaga H *et al.* Human thrombin plus 5 per cent ethanolamine oleate injected to sclerose oesophageal varices: a prospective randomized trial. *Br J Surg* 1989; **76**: 715–718.

53 Snobl J, Van Buuren HR, Van Blankestein M. Endoscopic injection therapy using thrombin: an effective and safe method for controlling oesophago gastric variceal bleeding. *Gastroenterology* 1992; **102**: A 891.

54 Fugii Y, Sugawa C, Ozawa C. Haemostasis activation during esophageal variceal sclerotherapy with thrombin in cirrhotics. *Ann Surg* 1991; **57**: 222–225.

55 Williams SGJ, Peters RA, Westaby D. Thrombin – an effective treatment for fundal gastric varices? *Gut* 1994; **35**: 1287–1289.

Baveno II Consensus Statements: The Endoscopic Management of Variceal Bleeding

David Westaby (Chairman), Kenneth Binmöller, Roberto de Franchis, Norman Marcon, Shiv K. Sarin, Claes Søderlund, Henk van Buuren and Gregory van Stiegmann

1   Endoscopic techniques should be carried out at the moment of diagnostic endoscopy and remain the treatment of choice for an episode of oesophageal variceal bleeding.

2   Banding ligation has replaced injection sclerosis as the optimum endoscopic treatment to prevent recurrent bleeding from oesophageal varices.

3   Intravarix tissue adhesive and thrombin appear to be effective agents for gastric varices of the fundus and cardia but require confirmation by controlled trials.

4   Endoscopic sclerotherapy should not be used prophylactically; new endoscopic therapies have not been established as a prophylactic measure to prevent variceal bleeding.

Transjugular Intrahepatic Portosystemic Shunt (TIPS)

Jaime Bosch

INTRODUCTION

Ten years ago transvenous intrahepatic portosystemic shunt (TIPS) was an experimental treatment. Today, TIPS is an established therapy for some of the complications of portal hypertension [1]. Progress in research and in clinical application has been very rapid, and has generated much enthusiasm among hepatogastroenterologists and radiologists. A good example of this enthusiasm is the increasing number of articles and presentations at medical meetings related to TIPS during the past years. Probably over 5000 TIPS have been performed during that time. Apparently, the moment is appropriate for trying to assess where we are, what is known about TIPS and what needs to be defined by further studies.

This is the reason why at this Baveno II workshop it was deemed convenient to put together a panel of distinguished investigators to try to clarify these aspects, and to reach consensus where possible. This chapter is intended to introduce the more important or conflicting aspects of TIPS. A substantial part of it has been possible thanks to the effort of the panellists, whose help is deeply acknowledged.

TIPSS, IPSS, TIPS

At the beginning it was TIPSS. After a while, it lost one 's' to become TIPS, which is not entirely adequate since to use a stent to construct the shunt is still mandatory – and nothing suggests that this will change in the near future. However, TIPS can be done – and sometimes is done – not using the transjugular vein approach; thus the T should be either dropped or should stand for 'transvenous' rather than 'transjugular'.

WHAT IS TIPS?

TIPS is an intrahepatic portosystemic shunt which is established using interventional radiology techniques. Haemodynamically, TIPS is almost identical to a small diameter ('calibrated') mesocaval or portocaval H-graft shunt, behaving as a side-to-side shunt. As such, it allows the reduction of portal pressure and the decompression of the liver, and is therefore appropriate both for the treatment of gastro-oesophageal variceal bleeding and of ascites (and of the Budd–Chiari syndrome) [2].

As a 'calibrated' shunt, TIPS has the potential to offer enough portal decompression to correct the complications of portal hypertension, while maintaining some portal liver perfusion (preventing a further impairment of liver function). By being a 'partial' shunt, TIPS has the potential of causing less encephalopathy than total shunts.

WHAT SHOULD BE ACHIEVED BY TIPS?

Obviously, the aim of any therapy is to cure or prevent the condition it is used for. Thus, we could state that TIPS should effectively correct and/or prevent the complications of portal hypertension. However, this should be done without causing too much harm. Therefore, the question arises about how much we should shunt with a TIPS, which in practice is substituted for how much we should dilate a TIPS, and what guidelines should be used when doing so.

Haemodynamic targets

From drug therapy studies we know that prevention of first bleeding from the gastro-oesophageal varices requires that the portohepatic gradient (PHG) – the pressure gradient between the portal vein and the hepatic vein or inferior vena cava – be reduced to 12 mmHg or below [3]. Thus, it seems sound to dilate a TIPS until the PHG is reduced to values $\leqslant 12$ mmHg. However, this is rarely done, and many centres adhere to a 50% decrease of the PHG, which is entirely arbitrary and without any scientific basis. Moreover, quite often the pressure gradient is calculated as the portosystemic gradient (PSG), using the right atrial pressure instead of the hepatic vein or inferior vena cava (IVC) pressure. This is important because all clinical correlations of haemodynamic measurements in portal hypertension have been established with PHG – not with the PSG. I strongly support continuing to measure the PHG (while I have no objection to measurements of PSG as well).

Another issue is the way of measuring the PHG. This should be done using appropriately calibrated pressure transducers, obtaining permanent tracings that allow its review whenever needed, and performing the measurements correctly (without having contrast dye in the catheters; before angiography; taking measurements in triplicate; avoiding the use of water columns, etc.). A golden rule is that accurate measurements can only be done if there is no hurry in obtaining them.

Portographic findings

Another common way of 'adjusting' TIPS is to observe the cessation of variceal filling on portography [1]. Again, there is no study showing if this is needed for an effective prevention of bleeding, or if by doing so, TIPS is no longer acting as a partial shunt. In addition, 'filling of the varices' at portography can be markedly influenced by the rate and pressure of dye delivery, and the site of injection (i.e. it is easier to demonstrate these collaterals after a splenic vein injection than injecting at the portal vein trunk). Therefore, there is also a difficulty in standardizing – and making objective – the findings of portography.

WHAT ARE THE ESTABLISHED INDICATIONS OF TIPS?

The potential indications of TIPS include the correction and/or prevention of all the complications of portal hypertension. TIPS has actually been reported to be successful in almost every case. However, there is not a single randomized controlled trial (RCT) demonstrating a clear-cut advantage of TIPS. Instead, there has been a tendency of accepting as established indications situations in which the benefit of therapy is reasonably suspected. These assumptions, however, are dangerous, inasmuch as they may reflect more the wishful thinking of enthusiastic physicians, rather than scientifically proven facts.

A list of the most commonly quoted 'accepted' indications and a list of those commonly thought to require confirmation by RCTs is given in Table 15. My personal view is to accept as established the indications in which TIPS is in fact the only possible therapy (i.e. the patient with advanced liver failure who does not stop bleeding from varices, despite medical, pharmacological and endoscopic therapy; or the Child–Pugh C patient having gone through three admissions for bleeding varices in 6 months despite sclerotherapy/banding and/or drugs) [4]. Even in these 'compassionate' situations, however, it may be that TIPS has nothing to offer (i.e. in the patient with a Child–Pugh score of 15). Thus, all the indications suggested probably ought to be subjected to RCTs. An effort should be made towards that aim, including the assignment of funding by public agencies and the encouragement of multicentre studies with realistic sample-size calculations. It is frustrating to verify that new therapies deserve less powerful trials than others that we know a lot more about.

Table 15 Indications for TIPS.

'Accepted' indications*	Suitable patients
1 Treatment of acute bleeding	Failure of medical and endoscopic therapy Child class C Gastric varices
2 Treatment of the Budd–Chiari syndrome	
3 Prevention of rebleeding from varices and portal hypertensive gastropathy	As a 'rescue' treatment after failure of medical endoscopic therapy Child–Pugh class C (but ⩽ 12 points) Patients on a waiting list for orthotopic liver transplantation
4 Treatment of refractory ascites	Non-terminal patients without organic kidney damage
5 Treatment of pre-hepatic portal hypertension	Patients without cavernomatous transformation of the portal vein
*Other:** 1 Ancillary therapy in the preparation for liver transplantation ('all comers') 2 First-line treatment of variceal haemorrhage ('all comers') 3 Prevention of first bleeding in patients at high risk (patients with grade III varices, red colour signs and Child–Pugh classes B and C) 4 Treatment of ascites ('all comers')	

* None has been firmly established by appropriate randomized controlled trials.

Special note

There is not a single study to support the use of TIPS in the preparation for orthotopic liver transplantation, which is often claimed to be an 'established indication'.

WHAT ARE THE RESULTS OF TIPS?

Tables 16–18 summarize the main findings of reported studies dealing with the results of TIPS in the treatment of acute variceal bleeding [5–9], prevention of recurrent bleeding [10–13] and severe or refractory ascites [14–21]. It should be noted that most studies are preliminary reports, that definitions of medically uncontrollable bleeding and refractory ascites are quite heterogeneous and may contribute to the heterogeneity of the results, and that the severity of the underlying liver disease varies markedly from one

Table 16 TIPS in the emergency treatment of variceal bleeding.

Reference	No. of patients	Child–Pugh class A/B/C	Length of follow-up (months)	Rebleeding during follow-up (%)	Mortality rate (%)
Sanyal et al. [5]	20	0/3/17	4	?	50
Barange et al. [6]	40	–/–/28	9	23	58
Jalan et al. [7]	19	NA	1.5	16	42
McCormick et al. [8]	20	1/7/12	NA	40	70
Casado et al. [9]	32	8/11/13	14	28	25

NA, not available.

study to another. I would like to call your attention to several important points.

1   The reported results are quite heterogenous – bigger and better trials will be required to clarify the real treatment effect.

2   The mortality may be quite high (much higher than expected) and correlates with the Child–Pugh score.

3   The success rate reported in these studies is lower than that achieved with traditional shunt surgery, especially when the follow-up is of more than 1 year, due to a very high incidence of TIPS dysfunction. This is due in most instances to the stenosis of the stent or of the hepatic veins, very often requiring repeated angioplasty and restenting. This is one of the major problems of TIPS, and is further discussed below.

4   The incidence of encephalopathy is also high – in the range reported for total stunts.

HOW DO WE KNOW THAT A TIPS IS WORKING PROPERLY?

When bleeding or ascites recur it is easy to conclude that TIPS is likely not to be working adequately. It is a bit more difficult to answer the question in the patient without complications. There is not even an agreement on what shall be considered a malfunctioning TIPS, and how and when this should be investigated. Doppler ultrasound (US) (preferably colour-coded) is claimed to be highly sensitive and specific. Unfortunately, this is not entirely true. Actually, Doppler US frequently rules out dysfunction of a malfunctioning TIPS or suggests a non-existent dysfunction. Other ways of diagnosis are not much better; an increase in the size of varices at endoscopy is very suggestive, but faces the problem of poor intra- and interobserver agreement. Portography is excellent to demonstrate occlusion of TIPS, but much less accurate in detecting haemodynamically significant stenosis. Pressure measurements

Table 17 Preliminary results of randomized controlled trials comparing TIPS vs. endoscopic sclerotherapy (EST) for the prevention of recurrent variceal bleeding.

Reference	No. of patients		Rebleeding during follow-up (%)		Mortality rate (%)		Length of follow-up (months)	Portosystemic encephalopathy (%)	
	TIPS	EST	TIPS	EST	TIPS	EST		TIPS	EST
Sanyal et al. [10]	40	39	25	20	28	10	12	23*	15†
Cabrera et al. [11]	29	29	21	57	18	18	14	29	14
Merli et al. [12]	23	23	13	30	13	9	7	39	9
Rössle et al. [13]‡	26	27	8	26	8	4	8	19	0

* 24 episodes.
† Six episodes.
‡ Esclerosis + propranolol.

Table 18 TIPS in the treatment of refractory ascites.

Reference	No. of patients	Child-Pugh class A/B/C	Resolution/ improvement (%)	Early mortality rate (%)	Overall mortality rate (%)	Portosystemic encephalopathy (%)	Length of follow-up
Ferral et al. [14]*	14	0/6/8	50	14	43†	36	2–18 months
Somberg et al. [15]	5	NA	100	NA	NA	NA	1–6 months
Pomier-Layrargues et al. [16]	19	0/15/4	79	NA	42	26	3–8 months
Ochs et al. [17]	36	–/–/30	93	8	36	25	NA
García-Villareal et al. [18]	12	NA	100	NA	NA	NA	NA
Benner et al. [19]	22	0/9/13	63	32	NA‡	NA	NA
Grangé et al. [20]	7	0/4/3	57	NA	29	43	NA
Gordon et al. [21]	26	0/12/14	69	NA	42	NA	7 months
Lebrec et al. [22]§ {TIPS	13	0/9/4	69	NA	83	8	1 month–2 years
{Paracentesis	12	0/8/4	33	NA	42	0	1 month–2 years

* Only study using internationally approved criteria to define refractory ascites.
† All five patients with a score > 11 died.
‡ All 13 Child C patients died or had OLT.
§ Preliminary results from a randomized controlled trial vs. paracentesis.
NA, not available.

across the shunt are likely to be close to a gold standard, but we do not know well enough what the safety level that we have to achieve is. Whether the 12 mmHg threshhold is also useful to define TIPS dysfunction has yet to be proven. As yet, there is absolutely no basis for the use of a 15 mmHg cut-off which is used in some centres.

We know that TIPS dysfunction is very common. We should probably be able to detect it easily and correct it before the appearance of clinical complications. The problem is that we do not know what we should look at, and when and how often. Probably it is adequate to have an early look at the TIPS (during the first week(s)) and repeat examinations at scheduled intervals (3, 6, 12 months, etc.). Even if this does not prove to be useful, it is the only way of collecting the information that we require to answer this question.

CAN WE REDUCE THE RISK OF TIPS DYSFUNCTION?

Over 50% of TIPS become malfunctioning after 6–12 months. This causes important problems because of the strict follow-up protocol required for detection of TIPS dysfunction before the appearance of clinical complications. Such an active surveillance markedly increases the cost and effort associated with this treatment. The mechanism of TIPS dysfunction is not known, which precludes the application of rational therapy to prevent it. This is an area of great priority for research, including the investigation of the mechanisms and of whether new stent design or drug therapy can minimize the risk of dysfunction.

WHAT SHOULD WE DO WHEN WE DETECT TIPS DYSFUNCTION?

Another problem yet to be solved is what is the best attitude when dysfunction is proven. Shall we dilate and/or restent all cases, or only those in whom there is total occlusion or a PHG > 12 mmHg? How many times should we restent a patient with repeated TIPS dysfunction? These are relevant questions since they can affect the efficiency of therapy, and also because of the cost of repeat stenting.

CAN WE PREDICT THE RISK OF ENCEPHALOPATHY? SHALL WE DO SOMETHING TO REDUCE IT?

A major drawback for any kind of portosystemic shunt is the development of portosystemic encephalopathy. TIPS is not an exception, and the encephalopathy rates of 10–30% reported are within the range observed with surgical shunts [2,23]. Although in most cases encephalopathy is mild, in one-fifth of the patients it is chronic and disabling, and may require closure or reduction of TIPS. Obviously, it would be helpful if patients prone to developing encephalopathy could be identified before TIPS. Since encephalopathy is influenced by the degree of shunting and of liver failure, it could be that measurements of both could help in identifying patients at a high risk of developing chronic, disabling encephalopathy.

Factors that appear to be useful in predicting encephalopathy are old age, diameter of stent (> 10 mm) and a history of previous episodes of encephalopathy. In these cases it may be adequate to institute some prophylactic measures, such as moderate dietary restriction and lactulose/lactitol administration in patients with constipation. It is important to instruct the patient's relatives so they can identify signs of impending hepatic encephalopathy and institute the appropriate therapy early.

WHAT IS THE FUTURE OF TIPS?

TIPS will find an increasing use in the treatment of portal hypertension, only if the following can be achieved.

1   A decrease in the incidence of TIPS dysfunction to 'reasonable' figures. Only about 20% of patients should develop TIPS dysfunction.

2   A reduction in the cost related to the procedure. Unfortunately, cost is an important issue. In reducing the cost of TIPS, it is more important to be able to prevent TIPS dysfunction than to have cheaper stents.

3   Demonstration in RCTs of its superiority over 'standard' treatments.

Acknowledgements

This work was supported by grants from the Fondo de Investigación Sanitaria FIS 94/0757. Diana Bird provided expert assistance in the preparation of this manuscript.

REFERENCES

1 Rössle M, Haag K, Ochs A *et al.* The transjugular intrahepatic portosystemic stent shunt procedure for variceal bleeding. *N Engl J Med* 1994; 330: 165–171.

2 Bosch J, Groszmann RJ (eds), *Portal Hypertension, Pathophysiology and Treatment.* Oxford: Blackwell Scientific Publications, 1994.

3 Groszmann RJ, Bosch J, Grace N *et al.* Hemodynamic events in a prospective randomized trial of propranolol vs placebo in the prevention of the first variceal hemorrhage. *Gastroenterology* 1990; 99: 1401–1407.

4 Bosch J, Bañares R, Bilbao JI *et al.* Derivación portosistémica percutánea intrahepática (TIPS). *Gastroenterol Hepatol* 1993: 16: 544–549.

5 Sanyal AJ, Freedman AM, Shiffman ML *et al.* Transjugular intrahepatic portosystemic

shunt for uncontrolled variceal hemorrhage in advanced cirrhotics at high-risk for surgery: a prospective study (abstract). *Gastroenterology* 1993; **104**: A985.

6 Barange K, Rousseau H, Vinel JP *et al*. TIPS as an emergency procedure in actively bleeding patients with advanced cirrhosis (abstract). *Hepatology* 1994; **20**: 46.

7 Jalan R, John TG, Redhead DN, Garden OJ, Finlayson NDC, Hayes PC. TIPSS vs oesophageal transection in the management of uncontrolled variceal haemorrhage (abstract). *Hepatology* 1994: **20**: 1061.

8 McCormick PA, Dick R, Panagou EB *et al*. Emergency transjugular intrahepatic portosystemic stent shunting as a salvage treatment for uncontrolled variceal bleeding. *Br J Surg* 1994; **81**: 1324–1327.

9 Casado M, Bañares R, Rodriguez-Laiz JM *et al*. Derivación portosistémica percutánea intrahepática (TIPS) urgente en el tratamiento de la hemorragia aguda de origen variceal (abstract). *Gastroenterol Hepatol* 1995 (in press).

10 Sanyal AJ, Freedman AM, Purdum PP *et al*. Transjugular intrahepatic portosystemic shunt vs sclerotherapy for prevention of recurrent variceal hemorrhage: a randomized prospective trial (abstract). *Gastroenterology* 1994; **106**: A975.

11 Cabrera J, Maynar M, Granados R *et al*. Transjugular intrahepatic portosystemic shunt vs sclerotherapy in the elective treatment of variceal bleeding (abstract). *Hepatology* 1994: **20**: 425.

12 Merli M, Riggio O, Capocaccia L *et al*. Transjugular intrahepatic portosystemic shunt vs endoscopic sclerotherapy in preventing variceal rebleeding: preliminary results of a randomized controlled trial (abstract). *Hepatology* 1994; **20**: 43.

13 Rössle M, Deibert P, Haag K, Ochs A, Siegerstetter V, Langer M. TIPS vs sclerotherapy and β-blockade: preliminary results of a randomized study in patients with recurrent variceal hemorrhage (abstract). *Hepatology* 1994; **20**: 44.

14 Ferral H, Bjarnason H, Wegryn SA *et al*. Refractory ascites: early experience in treatment with transjugular intrahepatic portosystemic shunt. *Radiology* 1993; **189**: 795–801.

15 Somberg KA, Lake JR, Tomlanovich SJ, Laberge JM, Bass NM. Transjugular intrahepatic portosystemic shunt for refractory ascites: assessment of clinical and humoral response and renal function (abstract). *Gastroenterology* 1993; **104**: A998.

16 Pomier-Layrargues G, Legault L, Roy L, Dufresne PM, Lafortune M, Fenyves D. TIPSS for treatment of refractory ascites: a pilot study (abstract). *Hepatology* 1993; **18**: 187.

17 Ochs A, Sellinger M, Haag K, Langer M, Blum U, Rössle M. TIPS: efficacy and survival in 36 patients with refractory and untreatable ascites (abstract) *J Hepatol* 1993; **18** (Suppl. 1): S59.

18 García-Villareal L, Zozaya JM, Nuñez M *et al*. Changes in sodium retaining systems after transjugular intrahepatic portosystemic stent shunt in cirrhotic patients with untractable ascites (abstract). *J Hepatol* 1993; **18** (Suppl. 1): S3.

19 Benner KG, Sahagun G, Saxon R *et al*. Selection of patients undergoing transjugular intrahepatic portosystemic shunt for refractory ascites (abstract). *Hepatology* 1994; **20**: 69.

20 Grangé JD, Boudghene F, Dussaule JC *et al*. Transjugular intrahepatic portosystemic shunt in cirrhotic patients with refractory ascites. Clinical efficacy and acute effects on aldosterone and atrial natriuretic factor (abstract). *Gastroenterology* 1993; **104**: A909.

21 Gordon FD, Stokes KR, Falchuk KR *et al*. Transjugular intrahepatic portosystemic shunt for the treatment of refractory ascites (abstract). *Gastroenterology* 1994; **106**: A900.

22 Lebrec D, Giuily N, Hadengue A *et al*. Transjugular intrahepatic portosystemic shunt vs paracentesis for refractory ascites. Results of a randomized trial (abstract). *Hepatology* 1994; **20**: 417.

23 Burroughs AK, Bosch J. Clinical manifestations and management of bleeding episodes in cirrhotics. In McIntyre N, Benhamou JP, Bircher J, Rizetto J, Rodés J (eds), *Oxford Textbook of Clinical Hepatology*. Oxford: Oxford University Press, 1991.

Baveno II Consensus Statements: TIPS

Jaime Bosch (Chairman), Gilles Pomier-Layrargues, Götz Richter, Oliviero Riggio, Plinio Rossi, Martin Rössle and Jean Pierre Vinel

1   Terminology: TIPSS, IPPS, TIPS. TIPS stands for transvenous intrahepatic portosystemic shunt.

2   Haemodynamics of TIPS. TIPS is very close to an interposition H-graft portacaval (or mesocaval) shunt. As such, TIPS allows the reduction of portal pressure and the decompression of the liver, and it is therefore adequate both for the treatment of gastro-oesophageal variceal bleeding and of ascites (and of the Budd–Chiari syndrome).

3   Targets. To have maximal efficacy without an exaggerated incidence of encephalopathy and shunt-induced liver failure, TIPS should be constructed as a small-diameter shunt. Shunt diameters >10 mm usually result in total shunting. Prospective studies will have to clarify this issue.

4   Uses of TIPS.

(a) TIPS can be used in the treatment of variceal bleeding which is uncontrolled by pharmacological and endoscopic therapy, both in the emergency situation and in patients with frequent repeated episodes of variceal haemorrhage, despite adequate elective treatment. TIPS can also be used in the management of the acute Budd–Chiari syndrome.

(b) All possible indications need to be tested in appropriately designed RCTs. These should have realistic sample size calculations and follow-up periods.

5   TIPS dysfunction.

(a) There is no agreement on the definition and diagnosis of TIPS dysfunction.

(b) Prospective studies are encouraged to provide the information required to reach consensus on this key issue.

(c) There is no effective way of predicting and preventing TIPS dysfunction.

(d) Detection of dysfunction should not automatically lead to restenting.

6   Encephalopathy.

(a) There is no way of accurately predicting post-TIPS encephalopathy.

(b) Post-TIPS encephalopathy is more common in patients >65 years old; when using large diameter stents; with a previous history of chronic encephalopathy.

(c) Disabling/progressive encephalopathy should be treated by reducing the diameter or by occluding the TIPS.

7   Requirements for establishing a TIPS programme

It is recommended for hospitals wishing to start a TIPS programme to fulfil the following requirements:

(a) written protocol with ethical committee approval;

(b) technical facilities (interventional radiology, ultrasonography, endoscopy, intensive care unit) and expertise in TIPS (minimal experience: 15 procedures) and in the management of the complications of portal hypertension; and

(c) defined follow-up protocol.

From Eck's Fistula to Liver Transplantation: a Critical Look at Surgery for Portal Hypertension

Alberto Peracchia, Giorgio Battaglia and Alessandro Baisi

INTRODUCTION

Although portal hypertension was first recognized and treated in the 20th century, the study and observation of the liver dates back more than two millennia, physicians of Hippocrates' time were able to palpate the liver and the spleen, and recognized jaundice and ascites. Moreover, Hippocrates understood that, in patients with jaundice, a hard liver was a bad prognostic factor. Studies were carried out by the famous Anatomic School at Alexandria: Erophilus (340–300 BC) accurately described the portal vein and the role of liver in nutrition, although knowledge of liver anatomy and physiology was very limited at that time. No improvement was made throughout the Middle Ages, but during the Renaissance, anatomic dissections became more common, and a better knowledge of anatomy became possible.

Studies of portal circulation began in 1543, with the printing of Vesalius' anatomic tables [1]. These were similar to a modern description, but, because of Galeno's influence, the portal trunk was divided into five different tributaries. Moreover, Vesalius understood that bleeding from haemorrhoids could be due to dilatation of peripheral portal tributaries, and he probably was the first to correlate gastrointestinal bleeding with a disease of portal circulation.

Two hundred years after Vesalius' observations, the link between gastrointestinal bleeding and portal circulation was recognized again: in 1762, Morgagni described a patient who died of gastric bleeding in whom 'polypoid concretions' of the splenic vein and huge dilatation of short gastric vessels were found [2].

A further hundred years passed before it was understood that collateral communications can develop between the portal vein and the vena cava through the short gastric vessels, the haemorrhoidal and abdominal wall veins, and oesophageal varices [3,4]. In 1872, Dusaussey published a thesis entitled 'Studies on oesophageal varices in hepatic cirrhosis', in which he maintained the obstruction to portal flow and development of collateral portocaval communications are due to hepatic cirrhosis (called 'gin liver' or 'brandy liver' by English authors) [5]. Supporting Dusaussey's hypothesis, Preble in 1900 reviewed the international literature and found 60 patients with liver cirrhosis in whom haematemesis was the cause of death. Oesophageal varices were found in 80% of these [6]. At that time, the sequence of hepatic cirrhosis, portosystemic communications, oesophageal varices, gastrointestinal haemorrhage and death, was evident. This prompted investigators to look for solutions aimed at reducing portal pressure and resulted in two approaches being identified: to reduce portal flow to the varices (by interrupting collateral circulation); and to improve the portal outflow.

IMPROVING PORTAL OUTFLOW

The first studies in humans in the early 1900s were based on previous experiments on dogs performed by a Russian surgeon, Nicolaj Eck. In Pavlov's laboratories he made a side-to-side portocaval anastomosis with interruption of the portal vein after the anastomosis, close to the liver [7]. The goal of Eck's studies was to treat ascites due to portal hypertension. Eight dogs were operated on, but only the last one survived for at least 10 weeks. Eck failed to complete his studies when drafted for military service, but his experiments were continued [8] and, in operated dogs, a central nervous system disturbance, called 'meat intoxication' and recognized as being due to shunting of intestinal blood into the systemic circulation, was observed.

For more than 20 years, the condition of portocaval anastomosis was only experimental. In 1902, the Italian surgeon Tansini published a new technique of end-to-side portocaval shunt with interruption of the portal vein and ligation of the hepatic stump of the portal vein [9]. One year later, during the XVI French Meeting of Surgery, the first portocaval shunt performed on a man was presented: it had been performed successfully by Widal in a patient with oesophageal varices and ascites [10]. The operation, carried out using the end-to-side technique, appeared relatively simple. After the operation, the patient did not bleed, but ascites relapsed after 6 weeks. The operation had been performed to treat ascites, but was successful in preventing bleeding. The patient survived about 40 months but died, probably from phlebitis. After the operation the patient had complained of central nervous system disturbances that developed after eating food with a high protein content. These symptoms were similar to the 'meat intoxication' observed in Pavlov's dogs. In 1893, Hahn and coworkers in Pavlov's laboratories noted that dogs did not develop 'meat intoxication' if the portal vein was interrupted before the confluence of the pancreatoduodenal vein [11]. Bogoras in 1913 [12], followed by Krestovsky in 1926 [13], anastomosed the superior mesenteric vein, before its confluence with the splenic vein, to the vena cava, in order to preserve an adequate blood flow to the liver. However, this modification could not prevent 'meat intoxication' because blood coming from the intestine was still entering the systemic circulation. In those years, the concept of maintaining an adequate blood flow to the liver was considered very important. De Martell in 1910 and Rosenstein [14] in 1912 performed laterolateral shunts in order to divide the portal flow between the liver and vena cava. However, a true improvement in the occurrence of 'meat intoxication' was not achieved by these first attempts; an improvement could only be obtained in the prevention of ascites. Moreover, the mortality rate of these operations was very high, probably due to the long clamping time necessary to perform the technically difficult side-to-side anastomosis.

Using a different approach, De Martell, Villard and Tavernier in 1910 [10,15] tried to reduce the amount of intestinal blood shunted into the systemic circulation by performing a small and distal anastomosis. This was done in a female patient, by anastomosing a tributary of the superior mesenteric vein to the right ovarian vein. The patient died 48 hours after the operation because of thrombosis of the shunt. Many other attempts at creating small shunts were performed in those years, but all were unsuccessful. Therefore, portocaval shunt became a very rarely performed operation in the following 30 years.

The surgical treatment of portal hypertension was considered again only in the 1940s, thanks to studies carried out in North America, and particularly in the Spleen Clinic at the Presbyterian Hospital of New York City, under the direction of Allen Whipple. It was now possible to perform long operations with blood losses, without fear of hepatic insufficiency and hypovolaemic shock. Whipple and Blakemore aimed at reducing portal hypertension with a haemodynamically efficient shunt. They studied both the end-to-side splenorenal shunt after splenectomy and nephrectomy and the side-to-side portocaval shunt. In 1945, Blakemore presented a series of 10 patients: five submitted to an end-to-end splenorenal shunt and five to end-to-side portocaval shunt using a vitallium prosthesis, as suggested 50 years before by Queirolo. The author's impression was that a portocaval shunt was more efficient than a splenorenal shunt in reducing portal hypertension and in decompressing oesophageal varices [16,17].

Mortality as a result of gastro-oesophageal variceal bleeding in patients with portal hypertension was so high that the main goal of portocaval shunts was to reduce portal hypertension and the incidence of bleeding, and therefore to improve survival. No attention was paid to long-term metabolic changes due to a total or near-total shunt of portal blood flow from the liver into the systemic circulation. Eck's observations about central nervous system disturbances, the so-called 'meat intoxication' in dogs, were not taken into account, even though in the same year a paper from Blakemore, George and Whipple reported the effects of Eck's fistula on haemoglobin and protein metabolism. After the operation the dogs resumed a normal life and achieved a good weight, but diuresis was decreased, jaundice appeared and protein metabolism became abnormal [18]. However, the supporters of the shunt thought that this was a low price to pay for a longer survival.

Meanwhile, suturing techniques were improving. In 1947, Blakemore anastomosed the porta directly to the cava, using Blalock's recently developed suturing principles. The surgical technique was now definitely established. The anastomosis between the portal vein and the vena cava was efficient in decompressing the portal system, with disappearance of oesophageal varices. The pressure difference between the porta and the cava was high, and the risk of shunt thrombosis low (11–18%). The enthusiasm for the initial success was so great that, consequently, surgical treatment of portal hypertension was adopted worldwide.

Although surgical treatment of portal hypertension was successful, medical treatment of liver cirrhosis and its complications has not improved over the past 30 years. Orloff noted that 'once a patient entered the hospital for treatment of cirrhosis, his chances of living for one year were about the same of those of a patient with acute lymphocytic leukaemia, and his chances of surviving 5 years were similar to those of most untreated cancers' [19]. On the other hand, the results of shunt operations were so good that some authors advocated the use of a portocaval shunt in patients with oesophageal varices as primary prophylaxis of bleeding. However, the results of four randomized studies [20–23] were so disappointing that prophylactic shunts were soon abandoned; the indications for shunt surgery were subsequently restricted to the prevention of rebleeding from oesophageal varices.

The pathophysiology of shunts was now evident. A large proximal shunt (portocaval or splenorenal) allows good decompression of the varices, but has a worse effect on liver function. A small distal shunt has fewer metabolic consequences, but has higher incidence of thrombosis and rebleeding. All shunts appeared haemodynamically similar, the main factor being the fall in portal pressure. Only the end-to-side portocaval shunt was different, because, by keeping a high pressure in liver sinusoids, it did not relieve ascites.

During the early 1970s, the concept of *selectivity* was introduced: its aim was to decompress the oesophagogastric varices without reducing portal flow. Inokuchi in 1970 [24] and Moreno Gonzales in 1974 proposed the anastomosis between the left gastric vein and the inferior vena cava with the use, if necessary, of a graft of saphenous or jugular vein [24]. In cases of hypersplenism, splenectomy, dissection of the tributaries of the splenic vein and ligation of the communications between the right and the left gastric veins were also performed. Gastrosplenic isolation was aimed at preserving blood flow to the liver and avoiding shunting of blood into the systemic circulation. Although the results presented by the author were excellent (encephalopathy 0%, rebleeding 8%), technical difficulties were high and the operation did not become very popular.

In 1967 Warren *et al.* [25] proposed a modified shunt aimed at selectively decompressing oesophageal varices while preserving the blood flow to the liver. The splenic vein was interrupted and the distal stump anastomosed end-to-side to the left renal vein in order to drain oesophageal and gastric varices through the short gastric vessels and the spleen. The right gastro-epiploic vein and coronary vein were ligated to isolate the portal circulation. However, the drawbacks of this operation soon became evident: (i) ascites was a contraindication to the shunt, which did not decompress the portal circulation; (ii) the procedure was not indicated in emergency oesophageal bleeding because decompression of oesophageal varices was slow; and (iii) gastrosplenic isolation was short-lived because, in a few months, portal blood was shunted again into the systemic circulation through the proximal splenic stump, the pancreas and the renal vein. Consequently, a few years later Warren proposed a modified operation with the dissection of the entire splenic vein from the pancreas and its interruption close to its confluence into the mesenteric vein. The splenic vein was anastomosed with the renal vein at the splenic hilum. Using this technique, a good liver blood perfusion was maintained long term, the incidence of encephalopathy was low and the long-term survival was improved [26]. However, this was a time-consuming and technically difficult operation, requiring great surgical expertise.

The operation proposed by Sarfeh *et al.* [27] was based on different pathophysiological principles. The porta was shunted to the cava with the interposition of a short 8-mm polytetrafluoroethylene (PTFE) prosthesis and the umbilical, gastroepiploic and left coronary veins were ligated to maintain a good inflow to the liver. An angiography was always performed in the first postoperative week and if the prosthesis was thrombosed a percutaneous thrombectomy was done. On the contrary, if collateral communications were still patent, they were closed by Gianturco stents. By choosing the size of the prosthesis accurately on the basis of portal flow measurements, and by ligating all collateral communications [28,29], Sarfeh could preserve a hepatopetal portal flow in 90% of patients, with an incidence of rebleeding of only 3.3% and of encephalopathy of 13% during a mean follow-up of 46 months.

DECREASING THE PORTAL INFLOW

When problems of shunt operations became evident, surgical procedures on oesophageal varices were proposed. The interruption of collateral communications sustaining varices can be done in different ways.

1   By ligating and sectioning all veins that reach and leave the oesophagus under the diaphragm and the proximal stomach (azygos–portal isolation).

2   By ligating directly the varices inside the oesophageal or gastric lumen (variceal ligature).

3   By interrupting the venous circulation in the oesophageal wall:

   (a) by means of a section of the oesophagus (oesophageal transection);

   (b) by causing the development of a sclerotic ring in the oesophageal wall;

   (c) by means of the resection of a small segment of the oesophageal wall (resection-anastomosis).

All the above techniques can be combined to achieve a complete devascularization.

The first direct operation on varices was proposed by Walter in 1929. It was the ligature of the left gastric vein and proved completely useless. Only in 1950 did Tanner develop an operation of true disconnection [30], later improved in 1961 [31]. The operation was based on the ligature of the lesser and greater gastric curvature vessels and of the short gastric vessels in order to interrupt the flow to varices in the proximal stomach and cardia. However, the isolation was disproportionate to the wide collateral communications present in portal hypertension, and the consequent incidence of early rebleeding was almost 50%. This operation was later modified by Schreiber and Bruer in 1964 [32] (subcardial gastric resection) and by Rinecker in 1975 [33] (mechanical transmural clamping), although results did not improve. The radical porta–azygos isolation proposed in 1963 by Torres [34] was based on a more correct pathophysiological principle. This operation included a wide oesophagogastric devascularization, the ligation and section of the left gastric artery, splenectomy to reduce the portal flow and direct ligation of the varices. In 1964, Hassab et al. [35] proposed the same operation but without ligation of the varices (gastro-oesophageal decongestion). These later operations gave excellent results: intraoperative mortality was 10% in elective cases and 12% in emergencies; the incidence of rebleeding was 7%. However, it must be considered that these results were obtained in patients affected by schistosomiasis.

In the 1950s Boherema [36] in Europe and Crile [37] in the United States developed a new technique for bleeding oesophageal varices. The oesophagus was opened through a left thoracotomy and the varices were directly transected by sutures. The indications of this operation were later extended to patients with portal thrombosis in whom a shunt could not be performed. Linton and Warren [38] in 1953 proposed this technique as a temporary emergency treatment before a shunt. The postoperative mortality was high, due to frequent suture leaks. In fact, the patients were usually of poor nutritional condition and the use of balloon tamponade before operation damaged the oesophageal wall, making suture leaks more likely. To improve these disappointing results, in 1954 Nissen proposed the extramucosal variceal ligation [39]. All these operations were efficient in emergency situations to control variceal bleeding, but the incidence of long-term rebleeding was high and they were therefore abandoned.

The first clinical application of the ligature and section of oesophagus on a metallic ring was made by Vosschulte in 1857 [40]. A silk suture encircling the oesophagus was placed on a prosthesis inside the lumen. This suture sectioned the oesophageal wall while a scar ring developed and interrupted the oesophageal varices; a splenectomy was also associated with this technique. In 1957, Boerema modified the operation by overlapping the oesophageal stumps above and below the ring in order to reduce the incidence of suture leaks. The inferior oesophagus was also devascularized to interrupt the blood flow to varices. Many other devices were later proposed, such as the Murphy ring, the Jabulay ring and the Prioton clips [41]. These techniques were easy to perform, but overall results were disappointing, with variceal bleeding relapse frequent and oesophageal stenosis occasionally developing.

In the 1960s Walker introduced the oesophageal transection [42]. This was an easy operation (section and immediate anastomosis of the thoracic oesophagus), with good bleeding control (relapse incidence of 15–30%), but some drawbacks soon became evident: (i) a thoracotomy was necessary; (ii) the oesophageal anastomosis could leak; and (iii) oesophageal varices relapsed and gastric varices were not treated. In 1976, Van Kemmel [43] suggested the use of autosuture staplers to transect the oesophagus. This operation could be done via an abdominal incision, with a subsequent decrease in the incidence of stenosis and leaks. This seemed a viable operation, safe and easy to perform, and very effective in controlling emergency bleeding, but bleeding relapses were frequent.

The only operation that seems able to provide control of bleeding both short and long term is the transection and paraoesophageal devascularization. This operation, originally described by Sugiura and Futagawa [44] was complicated and included thoracotomy and laparotomy, with up to 90 sutures on the oesophagus to achieve good haemostasis. The technique has since been modified in Europe to use a stapler to transect the oesophagus. The proximal stomach and 10–20 cm of the inferior oesophagus are devascularized, the operation being completed by a Toupet antireflux procedure.

At our institution, splenectomy is not performed in association with this operation, as originally proposed by Sugiura, because, in our personal experience, splenectomy increases the complication rate and does not improve short- and long-term postoperative results [45]. The excellent results obtained by Sugiura have never been reproduced in Europe. However, in our experience, this is one of the best operations currently available, especially in patients with prehepatic obstruction.

LIVER TRANSPLANTATION

Failures and high mortality of surgical treatment of portal hypertension are frequently due to liver insufficiency. The only surgical operation capable of curing the hepatic disease is liver transplantation, and this is therefore the only chance to cure the patient. Although today liver transplantation is less of a clinical challenge than in the past, it remains a difficult operation for the surgeon, for the anaesthetist and, obviously, for the patient. Moreover, transplantation cannot be proposed for all cirrhotic patients, not only because of cost and organ shortage, but also because it is not indicated in alcoholic and HBV-positive patients. Liver transplantation is the 'gold standard' for Child class C patients, but in those with fairly well-preserved liver function, endoscopic treatment or other surgery can provide results similar to transplantation. In our area, only one of 10 cirrhotic patients is a good candidate for liver transplantation.

CONCLUSIONS

Acute bleeding from oesophageal varices is undoubtedly the worst complication of liver cirrhosis. Although the sequence: cirrhosis → oesophageal varices → gastrointestinal bleeding has been recognized for more than 100 years, an ideal medical or surgical treatment is not yet available. All new therapies have given good results in selected groups of patients, but have failed in others. At the present time, liver transplantation, which would be the therapy of choice since it removes the cause of portal hypertension, cannot be proposed for all patients because of organ shortage, high costs and medical indications. Therefore, 50 years after the start of modern surgical treatment of portal hypertension, Whipple's pronouncement that: 'The problem of therapy for haemorrhage in cirrhosis will continue to be a serious one', is still valid.

REFERENCES

1 Vesalius A. *De Humani corporis fabrica.* Basileae, 1543.

2 Morgagni GB. *De sedibus et causis morborum per anatomen indagatis.* 9.111. Neapoli, 1762: 126.

3 Raciborski A. Histoire de decouvertes relatives au système veineux, envisagé dans le rapport anatomique, physiologique, pathologique et thèrapeutique depuis Morgagni jusqu'a nos jours. *Mèm Acad Roy Mèd* 1841; **9**: 447.

4 Sappey PC. Mèmoire sur un point d'anatomie pathologique relatif à l'histoire de la cirrhose. *Mèm Acad imp mèd* 1859; **23**: 269.

5 Dusaussey M. Etudes sur les varices de l'oesophage dans la cirrhose hèpatique. Paris: Thèse, 1877.

6 Preble RB. Conclusions based on sixty cases of fatal gastro-intestinal hemorrhage due to cirrhosis of the liver. *Am J Med Sci* 1900; **99**: 263.

7 Eck MV. K voprosu o perevyazkie vorotnois veni. *Voyenno-med J* 1877; **130**: 1.

8 Hahn M, Massen O, Nencki M, Pawlow J. Die Eck'sche Fistel zwischen der unteren Hohlvene une der Pfortader une ihre Folgen fur den Organismus. *Arch Exp Pathol Pharmakol* 1893; **32**: 161–210.

9 Tansini I. Diversion of the portal blood by direct anastomosis of the portal vein with the vena cava. *Gazz Med It* 1902; **53**: 323.

10 Vidal ME. Traitment chirurgical des ascites. *Presse mèd* 1903; 2(85): 747.

11 Hahn M, Massen O, Nencki M, powlow J. Die Eck'schje fistel zwischen der unteren Hohlvene und der Proftader und ihre Folgen fur den Organismus. *Arch Exp Pathol Pharmakol* 1893; **32**: 161–210.

12 Bogoras N. Ueber die ueberplanzung der vena mesenterica superior in die vena cava inferior bei leberzirrhose. *Munch Med Wochenschr* 1913; **60**: 1621.

13 Krestovsky W. Contribution a l'ètude du traitement operatoire des ascites cirrhotiques au moyen d'anastomoses immèdiates entre la veine cave infèrieure et la veine porte. *Presse Mèd* 1926; **34**: 1398–1400.

14 De Martel F. Lit l'observation d'une malade chez la quelle il ètablit une fistule d'Eck. *Rev Chir* 1910; **42**: 1181.

15 Villard E, Tavernier L. Suture ovario-mèsentèrique dans un cas de cirrhose du foie. *Lyon Mèd* 1910; **114**: 1113–1119.

16 Blakemore AH, Lord JW Jr. The technique of using vitallium tubes in establishing portacaval shunts for portal hypertension. *Ann Surg* 1945; **122**: 476.

17 Whipple AO. The problem of portal hypertension in relation to the hepatosplenopathies. *Ann Surg* 1945; **122**: 449.

18 Whipple GH, Robscheit-Robbins FS, Hawkins WR. Eck fistula liver subnormal in producing hemoglobin and plasma proteins. *J Exp Med* 1945; **81**: 171.

19 Orloff MJ. Emergency diagnosis and medical management of bleeding esophageal varices. In: Orloff MJ, Stipa S, Ziparo V (eds), *Medical and Surgical Problems of Portal Hypertension. Proceedings of the Serono Symposia, Vol 34.* New York: Academic Press, 1980: 386–398.

20 Jackson FC, Perrin EB, Smith AG, Dagradi AE, Nadal HM. A clinical investigation of the porta-caval shunt. II Survival analysis of the prophylactic operation. *Am J Surg* 1967; **115**: 22.

21 Resnick RH, Chalmers TC, Ishiara AM *et al.* A controlled study of the porta-caval shunt. A final report. *Ann Intern Med* 1969; **70**: 675.

22 Conn HO. Prophylactic portacaval shunts. *Ann Intern Med* 1972; **70**: 859.

23 Conn HO, Lindenmuth WW. Prophylactic porta-caval anastomosis in cirrhotic patients with esophageal varices. Interim results with suggestions for subsequent investigation. *N Engl J Med* 1972; **272**: 725.

24 Inokuchi K, Kobayashi M, Kusaba A. New selective decompression of esophageal varices by a left gastric venous-caval shunt. *Arch Surg* 1970; **100**: 157.

25 Warren WD, Zeppa R, Fomon JJ. Selective transsplenic decompression of gastro-esophageal varices by distal spleno-renal shunt. *Ann Surg* 1967; **166**: 437.

26 Maffei-Faccioli A, Gerunda GE, Neri D, Merenda R, Zangrandi F, Meduri. Selective variceal decompression and its role relative to other therapies. *Am J Surg* 1990; **160**: 60.

27 Collins JC, Rypins EB, Sarfeh IJ. Narrow-diameter portocaval shunts for management of variceal bleeding. *World J Surg* 1994; **18**: 211–215.

28 Marion P, Lapeyre D, De Bennetot M *et al.* Règulation d'une anastomose porto-cave par une vanne implantable animèe par une source magnètique. *Lyon Chir* 1971; **67**: 383–385.

29 Smith RC, Brown AR, Spencer PC *et al.* Percutaneous control of a portacaval H-graft: description of a new device and its initial clinical application. *World J Surg* 1990; **14**: 235–241.

30 Tanner NC. Haematemesis and melaena: an investigation of the place of surgery in its treatment. *Med Press* 1949; **221**: 9.

31 Tanner NC. Direct operations in the treatment of complications of portal hypertension. *J Int Coll Surg* 1961; **36**: 308.

32 Schreiber HW, Bruer H. Morphologische enzymologische und toxamische Fruhfolgen nach porto cavalen Anastomose. *Longenbecke Arch Klin Chir* 1963; **304**: 702.

33 Rinecker H. Indications bereiche maschineller nahtmethoden am gastrointistinal trakt: Operationsergebrisse dei 300 fallen. *Chirurgie* 1977; **48**: 241.

34 Torres UL. Rational basis of a new technique for treatment of portal hypertension. Operation Lemos–Torres–Degni. *J Cardiovasc Surg* 1965; **6**: 173.

35 Hassab MA, Younis MT, El-Kilanay MS. Gastroesophageal decongestion and splenectomy in the treatment of esophageal varices secondary to bilharzial cirrhosis. Anatomical and experimental studies. *Surgery* 1968; **63**: 731.

36 Boherema I. Bleeding varices of the esophagus, in cirrhosis of the liver and Banti's syndrome. *Arch Chir Nerl* 1949; **1**: 253.

37 Crile G. Transesophageal ligation in cases of bleeding esophageal varices. *Surgery* 1957; **42**: 583.

38 Linton RR, Warren R. The emergency treatment of massive bleeding from esophageal varices by transesophageal suture of those vessels at the time of acute hemorrhage. *Surgery* 1953; **33**: 243.

39 Nissen R. Blutende Oesophagusvarizen ohne portale hypertonie. *Schweiz Mediz Wochenschr* 1955; **85**: 187.

40 Vosschulte K. Place de la section par ligature de l'oesophage dans le traitment de l'hypertension portale. *Lyon Chir* 1957; **53**: 519.

41 Pioton JB, Laurent S. Recherche sur la dèconnexion portale de l'oesophage par ligature sur bouton de Murphy. *Montpellier Chir* 1970; **16**: 243.

42 Walker R. Esophageal transection for bleeding varices. *Surg Gynecol Obstet* 1964; **118**: 323.

43 Van Kemmel M. Ligature, rèsection segmentaire et anastomose à l'appareil PKS 25 de l'oesophage abdominal après hèmorragie par rupture de varices oesophaginnes. *Lille Chir* 1974; **29**: 80.

44 Sugiura M, Futagawa S. A new technique for treating esophageal varices. *J Thoracic Cardiovasc Surg* 1973; **66**: 677.

45 Peracchia A, Ancona E, Battaglia G. A new technique for the treatment of esophageal bleeding in portal hypertension. *Int Surg* 1980; **65**: 5.

Current Status of Surgical Treatment for Portal Hypertension: a 1995 Overview

J. Michael Henderson

INTRODUCTION

Previous workshops in the management of variceal bleeding in Gröningen in 1986 [1] and Baveno in 1990 [2] worked towards standardizing classifications of patients, bleeding events, diagnostic modalities, therapeutic strategies and methods in randomized trials. As a result of these workshops, these factors have been applied uniformly in studies of portal hypertension.

The goal of this session is to review the status of surgical options in the management of portal hypertension in 1995. This overview will update the reported surgical experience since 1990 as a basis for presenting consensus statements to the workshop. In the context of this meeting, surgical choices must be viewed as to how they fit in the overall scheme of other treatment options.

The surgical procedures available to manage patients with portal hypertension are as follows.

1   Liver transplantation.
2   Decompressive shunts:
   (a) total;
   (b) partial;
   (c) selective.
3   Devascularization procedures.

What is the current status of each of these methods?

LIVER TRANSPLANTATION

The indication for this procedure remains end-stage liver disease [3–5]. For many patients with portal hypertension, who present with one of its complications such as acute variceal bleeding, advanced liver disease is the aetiology of the portal hypertension.

For these patients a liver transplant is the only appropriate surgical option. The outcome for Child class C patients with variceal bleeding has been improved dramatically by liver transplantation, with a 65–75% 3-year survival. However, there are limitations:

1   many patients are not suitable candidates for transplant – active alcoholism, active hepatitis B, malignancy, severe concomitant disease;
2   the use of liver transplant is limited by donor availability; and
3   the high cost.

In the past decade the availability of liver transplantation has increased dramatically in Europe and the USA, and outcomes are greatly improved. In 1993, there were 3442 liver transplants in the USA and 3062 in Europe. The 1-year survival rates are between 80% and 90%, with 3-year survival 65–75%. As the indications for liver transplantation expand and results improve, there is an increasing discrepancy between the number of patients listed and those being transplanted. This will continue to widen. In the USA, the total number of donors has remained static for the past 4 years, despite the use of an increasing pool of 'expanded' donors.

The medical issues linked with liver transplantation for the management of patients with variceal bleeding and end-stage disease are clear. Transplantation relieves portal hypertension and controls variceal bleeding, while at the same time it restores liver function and corrects ascites, encephalopathy and the lethargy symptoms of advanced liver disease. Immunosuppression, with its associated risks of increased infection and malignancy and concomitant nephrotoxicity, is an acceptable price to pay for the above benefits. The medical efficacy of transplantation for appropriately selected patients is not disputed.

Areas of controversy currently being addressed in liver transplantation are high-risk groups and broader indications for transplant. Disease recurrence, and poor survival at high cost is an issue in patients with hepatitis B and C and patients with malignancies [6,7]. Transplantation treatment of the alcoholic is controversial and must be performed in conjunction with a full programme to manage the patient's total disease [8]. In the context of this workshop and variceal bleeding, the question can be asked if there are patients in whom the bleeding *per se* and not end-stage liver disease has become the indication for transplantation.

The average billed charge for a liver transplant in the USA is $280 000 for all charges related to hospital, physician fees, organ procurement, medications and follow-up for the first year following transplant [9]. The price war is raging and may well result in some cost reduction, in addition to limiting the number of transplant centres which must increasingly bear some of the risk in providing this high-cost care to patients.

DECOMPRESSIVE SHUNTS

Decompressive shunts provide palliative therapy for variceal bleeding. Decompression of varices controls bleeding in about 95% of patients, but the underlying liver disease is not corrected. However, decompression may be very appropriate for:

1 patients with presinusoidal portal hypertension and normal liver function;

2 patients with compensated cirrhosis, stable disease and adequate hepatocellular reserve; or

3 as a bridge to a transplant in some patients in whom it is estimated that their liver disease has $\geqslant 5$ years natural history before becoming end-stage.

Decompressive shunts for variceal bleeding fall into three categories.

1 Total portal systemic shunts which relieve all portal hypertension and divert all portal flow away from the sinusoids.

2 Partial portal systemic shunts which reduce portal hypertension to 12 mmHg and divert some portal flow away from the sinusoids.

3 Selective shunts which only decompress the spleen and gastro-oesophageal junction, maintain portal hypertension and thus maintain portal flow to the sinusoids.

Recent data on surgical shunts are summarized in referenced papers which include randomized controlled trials [10,12] and large consecutive series [13–18] of the different types of surgical shunts. The major outcomes are briefly reviewed below.

Survival

This is related to the severity of the underlying liver disease. Following total portal systemic shunt, Orloff achieved 65% 5-year survival in a predominantly alcoholic Child C population [10,12]. Partial shunt showed no significant difference in survival compared with total shunt, 75% at 2 years, in a randomized trial [11]. Distal splenorenal shunt (DSRS) in Child A and B patients can achieve a 91% 1-year and 77% 3-year survival [13]. A 60–92% 3-year survival rate after DSRS is reported in other recent series [14–17].

Control of variceal bleeding

This is $\geqslant 90\%$ with any of these surgical shunts, with slightly different risks with each procedure. Total portal systemic shunts, greater than 10 mm diameter, have excellent early control of bleeding: vein-to-vein anastomoses rarely thrombose [10,19], but prosthetic material has some risk over time of pseudo-intimal hyperplasia and thrombosis [20]. Partial shunts (8 mm diameter) appear to control bleeding as effectively as total portal systemic shunts, and in the available studies have not been found to have significant late thrombosis [11,21]. Distal splenorenal shunts have the greatest risk of variceal rebleeding in the first month as the decompressive pathway from the short gastric to splenic veins takes time to develop [22]. Late thrombosis of DSRS is rare, probably because this is a vein-to-vein anastomosis [23].

Encephalopathy

This occurs at different rates after the three different types of shunt. The most important variable in this is diversion of portal flow, a factor which increases the risk of encephalopathy. Thus, with total portal systemic shunts, encephalopathy occurs in 45–64% [11,18] and is severe in 10–36%. The lowest encephalopathy rates after total portal systemic shunt are reported by Orloff *et al.* [19]. In their population, encephalopathy falls from 55% before total shunt to 18.7% at long-term follow-up. They ascribe this low rate to their life-long programme of follow-up.

In a randomized trial, partial shunts had a significantly lower rate of encephalopathy at 21% compared with total shunt at 64% [11]. In uncontrolled series of partial shunts the rate of encephalopathy has been about 14% [21].

After DSRS, the overall rate of encephalopathy at late follow-up is approximately 15%. The incidence of severe encephalopathy is $\leqslant 5\%$. In a meta-analysis of the four prospective randomized trials comparing DSRS with sclerotherapy, there was no significant difference in the encephalopathy incidence after these two therapies [12]. This is probably the strongest available evidence that DSRS does not accelerate the rate of encephalopathy in patients with cirrhosis.

Cost

The cost of shunt surgery has been assessed by three groups [13,24,25]. These have looked at different components of charges. In summary, they show a hospital admission charge of approximately $23 000 [13,24,25] and total charges over 1–2 years to be approximately $35 000 [13,24]. It is of note that this later figure was similar to charges accumulated for sclerotherapy over 2 years.

DEVASCULARIZATION PROCEDURES

Devascularization procedures include a spectrum of 'direct' operations to treat varices. The components of these procedures are splenectomy, oeso-phagogastric devascularization and oesophageal transection. The classic Sugiura operation is a combined thoraco-abdominal procedure, performed in one or two stages which includes all these components. Lesser approaches have been associated with poorer results. Isolated oesophageal transection, an abdominal approach alone and devascularization without splenectomy have all been tried and have had higher rebleeding rates. Recent reviews of experience both in Japan [26] and outside Japan [27] help put the role of these procedures into perspective.

Survival

The operative mortality in a predominantly Child A and B group of patients in Japan has ranged from 3.5% to 12.4%. The cumulative 5-year survival rate (17% Child C) was 66% in this experience [26].

Studies performed outside Japan have shown operative mortality ranging from 0% to 25%, but insufficient data are available to comment on long-term survival [27].

One of the larger series from Orozco *et al.* [28] in Mexico documents good results in good-risk patients. In Child A patients they achieved an operative mortality rate of 12% and a 70% 5-year survival.

Rebleeding

The rate of variceal bleeding has been low in the major series in Japan, ranging from 1.5% to 6.5%. In experience outside Japan, in predominantly alcoholic patients, rebleeding rates of 20–49% are reported [27]. The experience from Mexico indicated a 6% rebleeding rate [28], more in line with the experience from Japan.

ENCEPHALOPATHY

Encephalopathy is lower than with any shunt procedure and is in the 7–12% range. The best available data on this are from the Brazilian controlled trial comparing total shunts, DSRS and devascularizations [29]. In this trial, DSRS and the Sugiura procedure had significantly lower encephalopathy than total shunt in this population with schistosomiasis.

SUMMARY

In the 1990s there are surgical choices for managing patients with portal hypertension. The decision on whether to proceed to surgery is dictated by the knowledge of the patient's disease and consideration of the risk/benefit ratio. Surgery should be considered in the context of a full programme for management of portal hypertension.

What operations are required in such a programme? Liver transplantation is mandatory, although the choice of other operations is based on available expertise. The data support the use of selective or partial shunt in preference to a total portal systemic shunt. Devascularization procedures work well in some good-risk patient groups.

REFERENCES

1 Burroughs AK (ed.), *Methodology and Reviews of Clinical Trials in Portal Hypertension*, International Congress Series 763. Amsterdam: Excerpta Medica, 1987.

2 de Franchis R, Pascal JP, Ancona E *et al*. Definitions, methodology and therapeutic strategies in portal hypertension. *J Hepatol* 1992; **15**: 256–261.

3 Starzl TE, Demetris AJ, VanThiel D. Medical progress – liver transplantation. *N Engl J Med* 1989; **321**: 1014–1022.

4 Henderson JM. Liver transplantation in portal hypertension. *Gastroenterol Clin North Am* 1992; **21**: 197–213.

5 Ringe B, Lang H, Tusch G, Pichlmayr R. Role of liver transplantation in management of esophageal variceal hemorrhage. *World J Surg* 1994; **18**: 233–239.

6 Samuel D, Muller R, Alexander G *et al*. Liver transplantation in European patients with the hepatitis B surface antigen. *N Engl J Med* 1993; **329**: 1842–1847.

7 Wright TL, Donegan E, Hsu JJ *et al*. Recurrent and acquired hepatitis C viral infection in liver transplant recipients. *Gastroenterology* 1992; **103**: 317–322.

8 Starzl TE, Van Thiel D, Tzakis A *et al*. Orthotopic liver transplantation for alcoholic cirrhosis. *JAMA* 1988; **260**: 2542.

9 Anders G. On sale now at your HMO: organ transplants. *Wall St Journal*, 1995; January 17.

10 Orloff MJ, Bell RH, Orloff MS *et al*. Prospective randomized trial of emergency portocaval shunt and emergency medical therapy in unselected cirrhotic patients with bleeding varices. *Hepatology* 1994; **20**: 863–872.

11 Sarfeh IJ, Rypins EB. Partial versus total portacaval shunt in alcoholic cirrhosis. *Ann Surg* 1994; **219**: 353–361.

12 Spina GP, Henderson JM, Rikkers LF *et al*. Distal spleno-renal shunt versus endoscopic sclerotherapy in the prevention of variceal rebleeding. A meta-analysis of 4 randomized clinical trials. *J Hepatol* 1992; **16**: 338–345.

13 Henderson JM, Gilmore Gt, Hooks MA *et al*. Selective shunt in the management of variceal bleeding in the era of liver transplantation. *Ann Surg* 1992; **216**: 248–255.

14 Maffei-Faccioli A, Geruuda GE, Neri D *et al*. Selective variceal decompression and its role relative to other therapies. *Am J Surg* 1990; **160**: 60–66.

15 Myberg JA. Selective shunts: the Johannesburg experience. *Am J Surg* 1990; **160**: 67–74.

16 Orozco H, Mercado HA, Takahashi T *et al*. Role of the distal splenorenal shunt in management of variceal bleeding in Latin America. *Am J Surg* 1990; **160**: 86–89.

17 Ezzat FA, Abu-Elmagd KM, Aly IY *et al*. Distal splenorenal shunt for management of variceal bleeding in patients with schistosomal hepatic fibrosis. *Ann Surg* 1986; **204**: 566–573.

18 Stipa S, Balducci G, Ziparo V *et al*. Total shunting and elective management of variceal bleeding. *World J Surg* 1994; **18**: 200–204.

19 Orloff MJ, Orloff MS, Rambotti M, Girary B. Is portal systemic shunt worthwhile in child's class C cirrhosis? *Ann Surg* 1991; **216**: 256.

20 Smith RB, Warren WD, Salan A *et al*. Dacron interposition shunts for portal hypertension: an analysis of morbidity correlates. *Ann Surg* 1980; **192**: 9–17.

21 Collins JC, Rypins EB, Sarfeh IJ. Narrow-diameter porta-caval shunt for management of variceal bleeding. *World J Surg* 1994; **18**: 211–215.

22 Richards WO, Pearson TC, Henderson JM *et al.*. Evaluation and treatment of early hemorrhage of the alimentary tract after selective shunt procedures. *Surg Gynecol Obstet* 1987; **164**: 530–536.

23 Henderson JM. Role of distal splenorenal shunt for long-term management of variceal bleeding. *World J Surg* 1994; **18**: 205–210.

24 Rikkers LF, Burnett DA, Valentine GD *et al*. Shunt surgery versus endoscopic sclerotherapy for long-term treatment of variceal bleeding. Early results of a randomized trial. *Ann Surg* 1987; **206**: 261–271.

25 Hermann RE, Henderson JM, Vogt DP *et al*. Fifty years of surgery for portal hypertension at the Cleveland Clinic Foundation: lessons and prospects. *Ann Surg* 1995 **221**: 459–466.

26 Idezuki Y, Kakudo N, Sanjo K, Bandai Y. Sugiura procedure for management of variceal bleeding in Japan. *World J Surg* 1994; **18**: 216–221.

27 Dagenais M, Langer B, Taylor BR, Greig PD. Experience with radical esophagogastric devascularization procedures (Sugiura) for variceal bleeding outside Japan. *World J Surg* 1994; **18**: 222–228.

28 Orozco H, Mercado MA, Takahashi T *et al*. Elective treatment of bleeding varices with the Sugiura operation over 10 years. *Am J Surg* 1992; **163**: 585–589.

29 Raia S, Mies S, Alfieri F. Portal hypertension in mansonic schistosomiasis. *World J Surg* 1991; **15**: 176–187.

Baveno II Consensus Statements: Surgery for Portal Hypertension in the Era of Liver Transplantation

J. Michael Henderson (Chairman), Giorgio Battaglia, Alvise Maffei Faccioli, Gianpaolo Spina and Vincenzo Ziparo

1   Liver transplantation is the treatment of choice for patients with portal hypertension and end-stage liver disease. The decision to transplant is based on appropriate selection criteria which may vary by disease.

2   Surgical shunts, and in selected cases devascularization, are appropriate therapy for patients with portal hypertension and preserved liver function who cannot be managed by endoscopic therapy and/or pharmacotherapy.

3   Where transplant is not available, devascularization can be an option in patients with poor liver function who continue to bleed through endoscopic therapy.

Efficacy and Efficiency of Treatments in Portal Hypertension

*Luigi Pagliaro, Gennaro D'Amico, Linda Pasta, Fabio Tiné,
Emma Aragona, Flavia Politi, Giuseppe Malizia, Aurelio Puleo,
Vittorio Peri, Adele D'Antoni, Rosanna Simonetti,
Giovanni Vizzini and Giuseppe Spatoliatore*

INTRODUCTION

The randomized clinical trial (RCT) is generally regarded as the most potent scientific tool for evaluating new treatments. However, limited attention has been paid to the process of translation of trial results into recommendations for clinical medicine, or to the correspondence between the efficacy of treatments as detected by RCTs and their efficiency in the unselected patient population in current practice [1].

This paper explores three related areas concerning the treatments for the prevention or the control of variceal bleeding in cirrhosis.

1   The correspondence and the temporal relationship between RCTs and therapeutic recommendations appearing in textbooks.

2   The clinician's choice between competing treatments in clinical situations where indications from RCTs are available or, conversely, in 'grey zones' [2] where no RCT-based sound evidence exists.

3   The behaviour of mortality in episodes of bleeding during the last decades, i.e. after the publication of a multitude of RCTs of treatments for the control of bleeding.

CORRESPONDENCE AND TEMPORAL RELATIONSHIP BETWEEN RCT'S AND THERAPEUTIC RECOMMENDATIONS IN TEXTBOOKS

Although we examined several treatments for the control or the prevention of variceal bleeding we show here only the three most representative examples.

Our general method was of summarizing the results of RCTs by a time-related cumulative meta-analysis [3,4]. This technique consists of performing a new meta-analysis each time a new RCT is added to the previous set of trials of the same treatment. Our selection was limited to the RCTs published as full reports in English.

We then compared the findings of cumulative meta-analysis with the recommendations of the same treatment appearing in 36 widely distributed textbooks (see Appendix) published between 1985 and 1995. The indications for treatments given in the textbooks were classified as follows: (i) 'not recommended', for the absence of conclusive evidence of efficacy, or for the risk of harmful effects; (ii) 'not mentioned', or 'mentioned', but without any explicit positive or negative suggestion; and (iii) 'recommended', for use in the generality of patients ('routine') or in a specific subset ('specific'). The examples we chose are dealing with sclerotherapy (EVS) for prevention of first bleeding ('prophylactic') and of rebleeding ('therapeutic') and with beta-blockers for prevention of rebleeding ('therapeutic').

Prophylactic sclerotherapy

Fifteen trials were reviewed [5–19]. Exceedingly favourable results were found in the first two trials. A statistically significant efficacy was detected by cumulative meta-analysis throughout the whole sequence of trials (Fig. 6). The effect size, however, substantially decreased since 1988 to the latest trial (1991). The direction of the therapeutic effect was negative in two large RCTs [9,19], with harmful results leading to the premature closure of the second [19]. A statistically significant benefit was only achieved in early trials with unusually high baseline bleeding risk (Fig. 6, lower panel). These contrasting results produced a highly significant statistical heterogeneity, increasing with the accumulation of trials. Prophylactic sclerotherapy was recommended in only one textbook scrutinized, published in 1985. In the others, sclerotherapy was not mentioned or, if mentioned, was often explicitly not recommended for current practice.

Thus, a clear contrast exists between the cumulative meta-analysis persistently showing significant efficacy of prophylactic sclerotherapy and the sceptic attitude witnessed by the textbooks. This can be plausibly accounted for by the contrasting results of the RCTs, with harmful effects in some of them, that were not detected by cumulative meta-analysis. The lack of a method for precisely quantifying the bleeding risk can be a further season for the cautious, conservative approach expressed by the authors in the related chapters in the textbooks.

Therapeutic sclerotherapy

Seven RCTs were reviewed [20–26]. The first RCT of therapeutic sclerotherapy admitting only patients with cirrhosis was published in 1982 [20] and showed a statistically significant benefit from the procedure. The effect size decreased until 1984, and then remained stable (Fig. 7). The direction of effect was favourable in all individual trials (i.e. odds ratios were below 1.0)

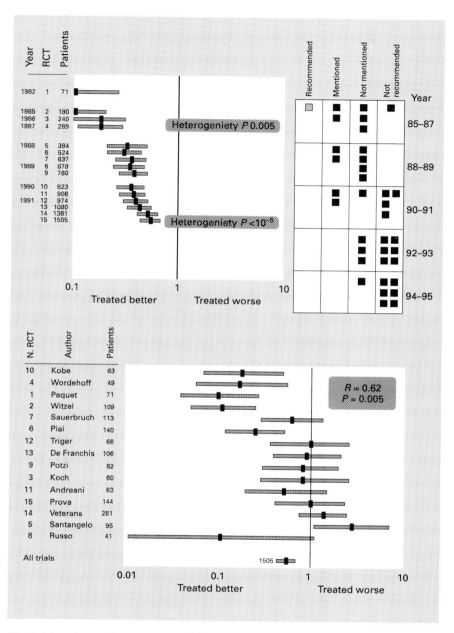

Fig. 6 Sclerotherapy for prevention of first bleeding. Upper panel: cumulative meta-analysis and recommendations of textbooks. Lower panel: standard meta-analysis according to the baseline bleeding risk in controls.

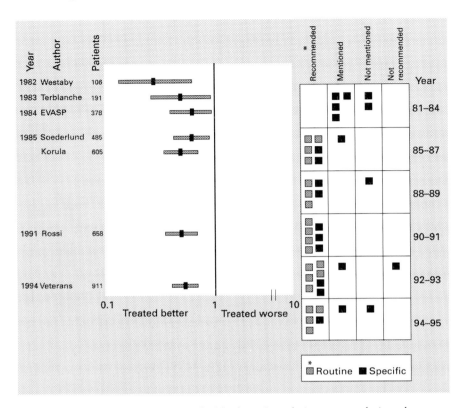

Fig. 7 Sclerotherapy for prevention of rebleeding. Cumulative meta-analysis and recommendations of textbooks.

except for one [21]. Recommendations of sclerotherapy were found in 30 out of 36 textbooks published since 1985. To assess when recommendations began to appear, we expanded our exploration to the years between 1981 and 1984, and found that sclerotherapy was mentioned, but not yet recommended, in four textbooks out of six.

Thus, the time interval between the first RCT showing the efficacy of therapeutic sclerotherapy and the appearance of recommendations in the textbooks was only 3 years, although two other RCTs published in 1983 and 1984 were inconclusive [21,22]. The early and general recommendation of therapeutic sclerotherapy in the textbooks is in contrast with the non-acceptance of sclerotherapy for prevention of first bleeding. A major reason for this difference could be the absence of harmful effects of therapeutic sclerotherapy in any trial, in contrast with the experience with the prophylactic use of the procedure. In turn, this could be due to the baseline risk, much higher and predictable for rebleeding than for first bleeding, that counterbalanced the potential complications of the technique.

Therapeutic beta-blockers

Nine RCTs were reviewed [27–35], one evaluating propranolol and atenolol [33]. A statistically significant efficacy was detected by the preliminary, pioneering report by Lebrec *et al.* in 1981 [27], and confirmed by the same authors in their final paper in 1984 [30]. Although three RCTs published between 1983 and 1987 [28,29,31] were inconclusive, cumulative meta-analysis showed persistent evidence of efficacy throughout the whole sequence of trials (Fig. 8). The direction of treatment effect was favourable in all RCTs (i.e. odds ratios were below 1.0 in all). Beta-blockers were recommended for prevention of rebleeding in one textbook in 1987 (see Appendix [31]), only mentioned or even not recommended in the textbooks published in 1988–89, finally reappearing in 1991. Since then, they were recommended in 10 of the 20 textbooks examined.

Overall, the acceptance of beta-blockers seems to be delayed in comparison with that experienced by therapeutic sclerotherapy. Since for both

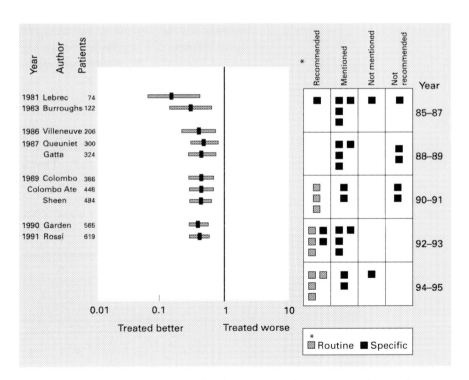

Fig. 8 Beta-blockers for prevention of rebleeding. Cumulative meta-analysis and recommendations of textbooks.

treatments there were inconclusive RCTs following the first favourable results, a different reason should account for the delay.

A plausible explanation may be the innovative quality of the treatment with beta-blockers, at a time when cirrhotic portal hypertension was mostly thought to be due to mechanical block, and unlikely to be affected by a drug.

THE CLINICIAN'S CHOICE BETWEEN COMPETING TREATMENTS

In order to obtain data about this issue we sent a questionnaire to three groups of clinicians with presumably scalar expertise in portal hypertension: the 49 participants in the Baveno II international workshop on portal hypertension (hereafter called 'Experts'), 123 members of the Associazione Italiana per lo Studio del Fegato (AISF) and of the Associazone Italiana dei Gastroenterologi Ospedaliere (AIGO) (hereafter called 'Specialists') and to 116 chiefs of Medical Departments of two Italian regions, i.e. Piedmont and Sicily (hereafter called 'Internists').

The questionnaire explored the options of these groups of clinicians for prevention of first bleeding and rebleeding and for control of bleeding. We have received so far 36 responses from Experts (73%), 46 for Specialists (37%) and only 15 from Internists (13%). Therefore, this preliminary report is limited to a selected set of responses from the first two groups.

Prevention of first bleeding in patients with large varices

Almost all components of both groups would prescribe a treatment, i.e. a beta-blocker, in patients with compensated cirrhosis (Table 19). This is

Table 19 Questionnaire question: would you prescribe a treatment for prevention of first bleeding in patients with compensated or decompensated cirrhosis and large varices? If so, which one? Values relate to the proportion (%) of responses received.*

| | Experts (n = 36) | | Specialists (n = 46) | |
| | Cirrhosis | | Cirrhosis | |
	Compensated	Decompensated	Compensated	Decompensated
Yes	91	59	93	51
Beta-blockers	82	41	78	22
Others (nitrate)	6	15	6	24

* Not all participants responded.

closely coherent with the sound evidence from RCTs that beta-blockers can effectively prevent bleeding in these patients.

A substantially lower proportion of responders from both groups chose to give a preventive treatment in patients with decompensated cirrhosis (i.e. with ascites, jaundice or encephalopathy). Several of those choosing to treat these patients would not give a beta-blocker (and preferred a nitrate preparation), particularly in the group of Specialists.

These options are not exactly coherent with evidence-based data. In fact, the data available show that patients with decompensated cirrhosis are at increased risk of bleeding [36], and RCTs or beta-blockers did not show harmful effects or decreased efficacy in decompensated disease [37,38]. Furthermore, the efficacy of nitrates for prevention of first bleeding is mostly supported by haemodynamic studies [39], whereas only one RCT has been published showing equivalent protective effect of nitrates in comparison with propranolol [40] in a sample including about 40% of patients with ascites.

Drugs for control of bleeding

The most interesting result of this section of the questionnaire was the choice of somatostatin or octreotide by about 50% of responders in either group (Table 20). This proportion is about three times higher than that of glypressin (only one responder from the USA chose vasopressin).

This discrepancy does not reflect the results of RCTs, which do not detect substantial differences between the two drugs (Fig. 9) [41–66]. Perhaps the low preference rate for glypressin can be accounted for by the experience of frequent and serious side effects with its analogue vasopressin. Although RCTs have shown a significantly lower incidence of side effects of glypressin in comparison with vasopressin with and without nitroglycerin [59–63], somatostatin is the only drug essentially free of side effects even when maintained for as long as 5 days [42].

Table 20 Questionnaire question: which drug would you use for control of bleeding? Values relate to the proportion (%) of responses received.*

	Experts ($n = 36$)	Specialists ($n = 46$)
None	15	4
Somatostatin/octreotide	44	58
Glypressin	13†	15
Either of the two	18	18

* Not all participants responded.
† Vasopressin + nitroglycerine used in one case.

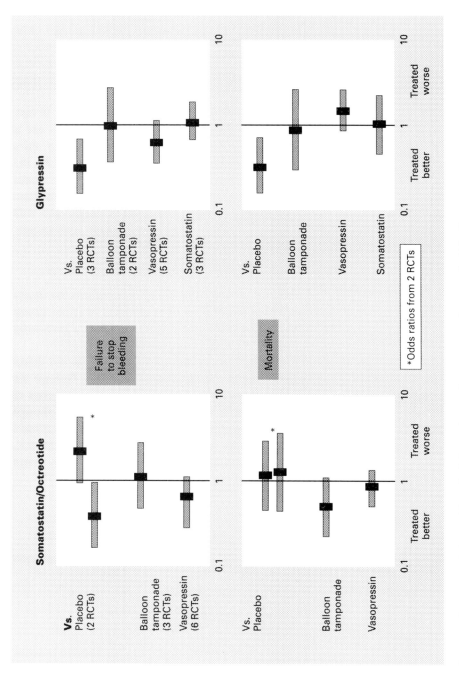

Fig. 9 RCTs of somatostatin/octreotide and of glypressin vs. other treatments for control of bleeding.

Treatments for control of bleeding after failure of drugs and sclerotherapy

There were some differences in the answers between Experts and Specialists (Table 21). In both compensated and decompensated cirrhosis, transjugular intrahepatic portosystemic shunt (TIPS) was chosen by a proportion of Experts about twofold more often than by Specialists; in contrast, surgery was chosen more often by Specialists than by Experts. It is of interest that TIPS was chosen by a proportion of responders as high as 68% and 56% among the Experts, respectively in compensated and decompensated cirrhosis, and by about one-third of the Specialists in either subset of patients. TIPS was indicated by some responders, mostly Experts, as an intermediate step waiting for transplantation.

TIPS clearly lies in a 'grey zone' as there are no available final reports of RCTs supporting its effectiveness for control of bleeding after failure of sclerotherapy.

Several reasons can explain the high preference rate given to TIPS in this context, i.e.

- preliminary favourable evidence from uncontrolled studies [67,68];
- pathophysiological similarity between TIPS and the highly effective surgical portocaval shunt [69,70], without the heavy perioperative complications of this latter procedure;
- absence or poor effectiveness of other therapeutic options in a desperate clinical situation.

The higher preference for TIPS among the experts was probably due to

Table 21 Questionnaire question: which treatment would you use for control of bleeding after failure of drugs and sclerotherapy? Values relate to the proportion (%) of responses received.*

	Experts (*n* = 36)		Specialists (*n* = 46)	
	Cirrhosis		Cirrhosis	
	Compensated	Decompensated	Compensated	Decompensated
None	3	9	7	18
Surgery	21	None	42	16
TIPS	68	56	33	36
OLT	3	20	4	15
Others†	3	9	7	7

TIPS, transjugular intrahepatic portosystemic shunt; OLT, orthotopic liver transplantation.
* Not all participants responded.
† Mostly repeated sclerotherapy or ligation.

their knowledge of early data from studies in progress and to the availability of TIPS in their units.

Prevention of rebleeding

Almost all responders in both groups were concordant in prescribing a treatment for prevention of rebleeding in patients with compensated disease (Table 22). The preference for this option in decompensated cirrhosis decreased more clearly among the Specialists. Sclerotherapy and an indifferent indication for either sclerotherapy or banding ligation were the most frequent options. Beta-blockers alone or their association with sclerotherapy were the following options, more frequently in compensated cirrhosis. Transplantation was frequently indicated by Experts for decompensated cirrhosis, whereas TIPS was indicated as an intermediate step towards liver transplantation by a few Experts.

Several points deserve comment.

1   The high preference rate for sclerotherapy and beta-blockers is coherent with the RCTs showing an equivalent efficacy of the two treatments [71]. However, the decrease of options for beta-blockers in decompensated patients again seems to indicate that these drugs are believed to be less effective or potentially harmful in advanced cirrhosis, although no data support this impression.

2   The frequent option of experts for banding ligation as an equivalent of

Table 22 Questionnaire question: would you prescribe a treatment for prevention of rebleeding in patients with compensated or decompensated cirrhosis? If so, which one? Values relate to the proportion (%) of responses received.*

| | Experts ($n = 36$) | | Specialists ($n = 46$) | |
| | Cirrhosis | | Cirrhosis | |
	Compensated	Decompensated	Compensated	Decompensated
Yes	94	88	91	71
Beta-blockers	24	15	27	13
Sclerotherapy	12	21	11	33
Sclerotherapy or banding ligation	26	29	16	2
Sclerotherapy or beta-blockers	18	3	27	13
OLT	3	21	0	7
Others	9	0	2	2

OLT, orthotopic liver transplantation.
* Not all participants responded.

sclerotherapy can be due to the interest for a new technique that appears to have a lower complication rate. The RCT-based evidence of this advantage, however, is still limited [72].

3   The frequent combination of beta-blockers with sclerotherapy is in agreement with a meta-analysis showing a reduced rebleeding incidence in patients receiving the combined treatment, although with some intertrial heterogeneity [73].

THE BEHAVIOUR OF MORTALITY IN EPISODES OF BLEEDING

We investigated the mortality in episodes of bleeding throughout the last decades. Our aim was to assess whether there was an improvement of prognosis over time. We first compared the 6-week (or in-hospital) mortality in nine 'old' cohort studies published between 1959 and 1974 with the mortality in controls not receiving specific treatments in seven RCTs published between 1982 and 1990 [74]. As shown in Fig. 10, there was a decrease in mortality from about 70% to about 35%. A potential bias of this comparison is the selection of good-risk patients in RCTs [75]. Therefore, we assessed mortality in 52 RCTs of non-surgical treatments for control of bleeding since before 1981 to after 1992 (Fig. 11). Assuming that any progress in the management of bleeding should result in a benefit for both

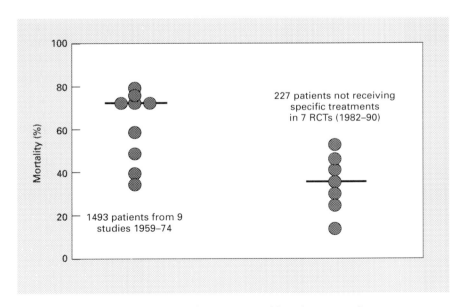

Fig. 10 Short-term mortality in bleeding patients: 'old' and recent studies.

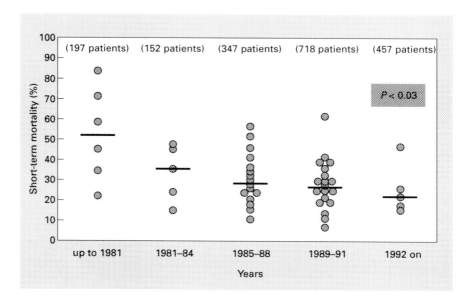

Fig. 11 Six-week or in-hospital mortality in 52 RCTs of treatments for variceal bleeding, including patients receiving both the experimental treatments and controls.

treated patients and controls, we assessed global mortality in the whole trial population. A statistically significant decrease in mortality was found. Finally, in order to re-evaluate these results in an unselected population of consecutive patients, we assessed mortality in the whole series of 350 patients admitted for a first episode of bleeding to our department between 1981 and 1990 (Fig. 12), again detecting a statistically significant decrease in mortality.

Since all treatments used for control of bleeding were previously assessed by RCTs, these findings show how the generalization of trial results can benefit patients in clinical practice.

There is also evidence that some changes occurring in the management of liver disease have improved mortality, without a substantial contribution of RCTs. A well-documented example is the improved survival of primary biliary cirrhosis achieved by liver transplantation [76]. Here we show that the survival rate of spontaneous bacterial peritonitis (SBP) increased in the last decades, before the publication of the few RCTs carried out in this area (Fig. 13).

This improvement in survival may be partly due to the inclusion in recent studies of mildly symptomatic or asymptomatic forms, not identified in early studies. However, it is sufficiently large to authorize the inference that survival rate really increased.

The factors determining the improvement of survival in SBP could be plausibly identified as follows:

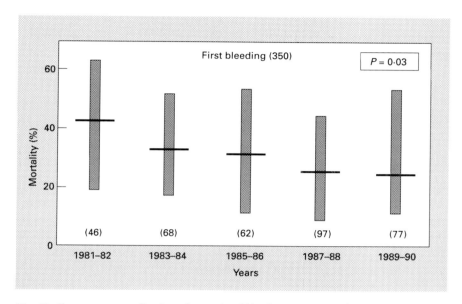

Fig. 12 Short-term mortality from first variceal bleeding in a series of consecutive patients (V. Cervello Hospital). Mean values and 95% CI.

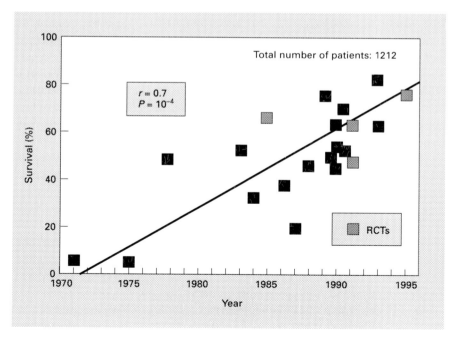

Fig. 13 Survival of patients in 21 studies of spontaneous bacterial peritonitis (SBP) in cirrhosis according to the year of publication.

1   the recognition in the 1970s and early 1980s of SBP as a frequent and life-threatening complication of ascitic cirrhosis, that led to the use of systematic paracentesis when suspecting SBP;
2   the identification of neutrophil count as a reliable diagnostic marker, leading to earlier treatment; and
3   the growing multiplicity of well-tolerated antibiotics highly active against Gram-negative bacteria, most frequently causing SBP.

FINAL REMARKS AND SPECULATIONS

Therapeutic recommendations in textbooks can be influenced by factors not reflected by cumulative meta-analysis. As shown for prophylactic scler-otherapy, cumulative meta-analysis can fail to detect intertrial heterogeneity, and particularly harmful treatment effects in individual trials. Authors of therapeutic recommendations in textbooks can perceive these data and adopt a (reasonably) cautious, conservative approach.

The wrong estimate of a low prior probability of pharmacological activity on cirrhotic portal hypertension is a plausible explanation for the delayed acceptance of therapeutic beta-blockers in textbooks. Perhaps a more accurate estimate of prior probability and a bayesian approach to the design and evaluation of RCTs [77] could be helpful for clinicians translating trial results into practice.

Overall, the therapeutic options of clinicians were most often supported by RCT-based evidence. Other influences, however, were also of importance.
•   The ancient warning *primum non nocere* probably prompted the high preference rate given to somatostatin/octreotide for the control of bleeding. Somatostatin/octreotide have a very safe profile, whereas in using the alternative drug glypressin there is a continued reminder of the serious and frequent side effects of its analogue vasopressin.
•   The high preference rate of TIPS for uncontrolled bleeding emphasizes the role of three factors generally determinant for medical decision making in the absence of RCT-based indications. These are: (i) a sound pathophysiological rationale; (ii) the severity of spontaneous prognosis; and (iii) the lack of alternative therapeutic options.

In conclusion, the responses to the questionnaire confirm that clinicians' therapeutic decisions depend on a complex interplay of factors, including RCT-based evidence, fear of side effects of treatments, severity of spontaneous prognosis and non-availability of other options.

Finally, the reduction of the mortality in episodes of bleeding seems to be due to generalization of treatments detected by RCTs as the most effective for the control of bleeding. Whereas this illustrates the importance of RCTs, the examples of SBP (and of transplantation in several liver diseases) shows that the continuous improvement in health care also depends on other factors such as the recognition of new syndromes and of their course, diagnostic advances and the discovery of new treatments.

Acknowledgements

The authors are indebted to Mrs Clara Profeta and Mr Antonio Lino, for their invaluable secretarial assistance.

REFERENCES

1 Eddy DM. Clinical policies and the quality of clinical practice. N Engl J Med 1982; 307: 343–347.

2 Naylor CD. Grey zones of clinical practice. Some limits to evidence-based medicine. Lancet 1955; 345: 840–842.

3 Antman EM, Lau J, Kupelnick B, Mosteller F, Chalmers T. A comparison of results of meta-analyses of randomized control trials and recommendations of clinical experts. Treatments for myocardial infarction. JAMA 1991; 268: 240–248.

4 Lau J, Schmid CH, Chalmers TC. Cumulative meta-analyses of clinical trials build evidence for exemplary medical care. J Clin Epidemiol 1995; 48: 45–57.

5 Paquet HJ. Prophylactic endoscopic sclerosing treatment of the esophageal wall in varices: a prospective controlled randomized trial. Endoscopy 1982; 14: 4–5.

6 Witzel L, Wolbergs E, Merki H. Prophylactic endoscopic sclerotherapy of oesophageal varices: a prospective controlled trial. Lancet 1985; i: 773–775.

7 Koch, Henning H, Grimm H, Sohendra N. Prophylactic sclerosing of esophageal varices: results of a prospective controlled study. Endoscopy 1986; 18: 40–43.

8 Wordehoff D, Spech HJ. Prophylaktische oesophagusvarizen sklerosierung. Dtsch Med Wochenschr 1987; 112: 947–951.

9 Santangelo WC, Dueno MI, Estes BL, Krejs GJ. Prophylactic sclerotherapy of large esopageal varices. N Engl J Med 1988; 318: 814–818.

10 Piai G, Cipolletta L, Claar M et al. Prophylactic sclerotherapy of high-risk esopageal varices: results of a multicentric prospective controlled trial. Hepatology 1988; 8: 1495–1500.

11 Sauerbruch T, Wotzka R, Kopcke W et al. Prophylactic sclerotherapy before the first episode of variceal hemorrage in patients with cirrhosis. N Engl J Med 1988; 319: 8–14.

12 Russo A, Giannone G, Magnano A, Passanisi G, Longo C. Prophylactic sclerotherapy in nonalcoholic liver cirrhosis: preliminary results of a prospective controlled randomized trial. World J Surg 1989; 13: 149–153.

13 Pötzi R, Bauer P, Reichel W, Kerstan E, Renner F, Gangl A. Prophylactic endoscopic sclerotherapy of oesophageal varices in liver cirrhosis. A multicentre prospective controlled randomized trial in Vienna. Gut 1989; 30: 873–879.

14 Kobe VE, Zipprich B, Schentke KU, Nilius R. Prophylactic endoscopic sclerotherapy of esophageal varices. A prospective randomized trial. Endoscopy 1990; 22: 245–248.

15 Andreani T, Poupon RE, Balkau B et al. Preventive therapy of first gastrointestinal bleeding in patients with cirrhosis: results of a controlled trial comparing propranolol, endoscopic sclerotherapy and placebo. Hepatology 1990; 12: 1413–1419.

16 The PROVA Study Group. Prophylaxis of first hemorrhage from oesophageal varices

by sclerotherapy, propranolol or both in cirrhotic patients. A randomized multicenter trial. *Hepatology* 1991; **14**: 1016–1024.

17 Triger DR, Smart HL, Hosking SW, Johnson AG. Prophylactic sclerotherapy for esopageal varices: long term results of a single-center trial. *Hepatology* 1991; **13**: 117–123.

18 de Franchis R, Primignani M, Rizzi PM *et al.* Prophylactic sclerotherapy (ST) in high risk cirrhotics selected by endoscopic criteria. A multicenter randomized controlled trial. *Gastroenterology* 1991; **101**: 1087–1093.

19 The Veterans Affairs Cooperative Variceal Sclerotherapy Group. Prophylactic sclerotherapy for esophageal varices in alcoholic liver disease: a randomized, single-blind, multicenter clinical trial. *N Engl J Med* 1991; **324**: 1779–1784.

20 Westaby D, MacDougall BR, Williams R. Improved survival following sclerotherapy for esophageal varices: final analysis of a controlled trial. *Hepatology* 1985; **5**: 827–830.

21 Terblanche J, Bornman PC, Kahn D, Jonker MA, Campbell JAH, Kirsch R. Failure of repeated injection sclerotherapy to improve long term survival after oesophageal variceal bleeding. A five-year prospective controlled clinical trial. *Lancet* 1983; **II**: 1328–1332.

22 The Copenhagen Esophageal Varices Sclerotherapy Project. Sclerotherapy after first variceal hemorrhage in cirrhosis. A randomized multicenter trial. *N Engl J Med* 1984; **311**: 1594–1600.

23 Söderlund C, Ihre T. Endoscopic sclerotherapy versus conservative management of bleeding esophageal varices. *Acta Chir Scand* 1985; **151**: 449–456.

24 Korula J, Balart LA, Radvan G, Zweiban BE, Larson AW, Kao HW. A prospective randomized controlled trial of chronic esophageal variceal sclerotherapy. *Hepatology* 1985; **5**: 584–589.

25 Rossi V, Calès P, Pascal B *et al.* Prevention of recurrent variceal bleeding in alcoholic cirrhotic patients: prospective controlled trial of propranolol and sclerotherapy. *J Hepatol* 1991; **12**: 283–289.

26 Veterans Affairs Cooperative Variceal Sclerotherapy Group. Sclerotherapy for male alcoholic cirrhotic patients who have bled from esophageal varices: results of a randomized, multicenter clinical trial. *Hepatology* 1994; **20**: 618–625.

27 Lebrec D, Poynard T, Hillon P *et al.* Propranolol for prevention of recurrent gastrointestinal bleeding in patients with cirrhosis. A controlled study. *N Engl J Med* 1981; **305**: 1371–1374.

28 Burroughs AK, Jenkins WJ, Sherlock S *et al.* Controlled trial of propranolol for the prevention of recurrent variceal hemorrhage in patients with cirrhosis. *N Engl J Med* 1983; **309**: 1539–1542.

29 Villeneuve JP, Pomier-Layrargues G, Infante-Rivard C *et al.* Propranolol for the prevention of recurrent variceal hemorrhage: a controlled trial. *Hepatology* 1986; **6**: 1239–1243.

30 Lebrec D, Poynard T, Bernuau J *et al.* A randomized controlled study of propranolol for prevention of recurrent gastrointestinal bleeding in patients with cirrhosis: a final report. *Hepatology* 1984; **4**: 355–358.

31 Queuniet AM, Czernichow P, Lerebours E, Ducrotte P, Tranvouez JL, Colin R. Etude controle du propranolol dans la prévention des récidives hémorragiques chez les patients cirrhotiques. *Gastroenterol Clin Biol* 1987; **11**: 41–47.

32 Gatta A, Merkel C, Sacerdoti D *et al.* Nadolol for prevention of variceal rebleeding in cirrhosis: a controlled clinical trial. *Digestion* 1987; **37**: 22–28.

33 Colombo M, de Franchis R, Tommasini M, Sangiovanni A, Dioguardi N. Beta-Blockade prevents recurrent gastrointestinal bleeding in well-compensated patients with alcoholic cirrhosis: a multicenter randomized controlled trial. *Hepatology* 1989; **9**: 433–438.

34 Sheen IS, Chen TY, Liaw YF. Randomized controlled study of propranolol for the prevention of recurrent esophageal varices bleeding in patients with cirrhosis. *Liver* 1989; **9**: 1–5.

35 Garden OJ, Mills PR, Birnie GG, Murray GD, Carter DC. Propranolol in the prevention of recurrent variceal hemorrhage in cirrhotic patients. *Gastroenterology* 1990; **98**: 185–190.

36 The North Italian Endoscopic Club for the Study and Treatment of Esophageal Varices. Prediction of the first variceal hemorrhage in patients with cirrhosis of the liver and esophageal varices. A prospective multicenter study. *N Engl J Med* 1988; **319**: 983–989.

37 Pagliaro L, D'Amico G, Sörensen TIA *et al.* Prevention of first bleeding in cirrhosis. A meta-analysis of randomized trials of nonsurgical treatment. *Ann Intern Med* 1992; **117**: 59–70.

38 Poynard T, Cales P, Pasta L *et al.* Beta-adrenergic-antagonists in the prevention of first gastrointestinal bleeding in patients with cirrhosis and oesophageal varices. An analysis of data and prognostic factors in 589 patients from four randomized clinical trial. *N Engl J Med* 1991; **324**: 1532–1538.

39 Garcia-Pagan JC, Feu F, Navasa M *et al.* Long-term haemodynamic effects of isosorbide 5-mononitrate in patients with cirrhosis and portal hypertension. *J Hepatol* 1990; **11**: 189–195.

40 Angelico M, Carli L, Piat C *et al.* Isosorbide-5-mononitrate versus propranolol in the prevention of first bleeding in cirrhosis. *Gastroenterology* 1993; **104**: 1460–1465.

41 Valenzuela JE, Schubert T, Fogel MR *et al.* A multicenter, randomized, double-blind trial of somatostatin in the management of acute hemorrhage from esopageal varices. *Hepatology* 1989; **10**: 958–961.

42 Burroughs AK, McCormick A, Hughes MD, Sprengers D, D'Heygere F, McIntyre N. Randomized, double-blind, placebo-controlled trial of somatostatin for variceal bleeding. Emergency control and prevention of early variceal rebleeding. *Gastroenterology* 1990; **99**: 1388–1395.

43 McKee R. A study of octreotide in oesophageal varices. *Digestion* 1990; **45**: 60–65.

44 Jaramillo JL, de la Mata M, Mio G, Costàn G, Gomez-Camacho F. Somatostatin versus Sengstaken balloon tamponade for primary haemostasis of bleeding esophageal varices. *J Hepatol* 1991; **12**: 100–105.

45 Avgerinos A, Klonis C, Rekoumis G, Gouma P, Papedimitriou N. Controlled trial of somatostatin and balloon tamponade in bleeding esophageal varices. *J Hepatol* 1991; **13**: 78–83.

46 Kravetz D, Bosch J, Teres J, Bruix J, Rimola A, Rodes J. Comparison of intravenous somatostatin and vasopressin infusion in treatment of acute variceal hemorrhage. *Hepatology* 1984; **4**: 442–446.

47 Jenkins SA, Baxter JN, Corbett WA, Devitt P, Ware J, Shields R. A prospective randomized controlled clinical trial comparing somatostatin and vasopressin in controlling acute variceal haemorrhage. *Br Med J* 1985; **290**: 275–278.

48 Bagarani M, Albertini V, Anza M *et al.* Effect of somatostatin in controlling bleeding from esophageal varices. *Ital J Surg Sci* 1987; **17**: 21–26.

49 Cardona C, Vida F, Balanzo J, Cusso X, Farre A, Guarner C. Eficacia terapéutica de la

somatostatina versus vasopressina más nitroglicerina en la hemorragia activa por varices esofagogastrica. *Gastroenterol Hepatol* 1989; **12**: 30–34.

50 Hsia HC, Lee FY, Tsai YT *et al.* Comparison of somatostatin and vasopressin in the control of acute esophageal variceal hemorrhage. A randomized, controlled study. *Chinese J Gastroenterol* 1990; **7**: 71–78.

51 Saari A, Klvilaakso E, Inberg M *et al.* Comparison of somatostatin and vasopressin in bleeding esophageal varices. *Am J Gastroenterol* 1990; **85**: 804–807.

52 Rodriguez-Moreno F, Santolaria F, Glez-Reimers E *et al.* A randomized trial of somatostatin vs vasopressin plus nitroglycerin in the treatment of acute variceal bleeding. *J Hepatol* 1991; **13**(2): S162.

53 Hwang JS, Lin CH, Chang CF *et al.* A randomized controlled trial comparing octreotide and vasopressin in the control of acute esophageal variceal bleeding. *J Hepatol* 1992; **16**: 320–325.

54 Walker S, Stiehl A, Raedsch R, Kommerell B. Terlipressin in bleeding esophageal varices. A placebo controlled double-blind study. *Hepatology* 1986; **6**: 112–115.

55 Freeman JG, Cobden MD, Record CO. Placebo-controlled trial of terlipressin (glypressin) in the management of acute variceal bleeding. *J Clin Gastroenterol* 1989; **11**: 58–60.

56 Söderlund C, Magnusson I, Torngren S, Lundell L. Terlipressin (triglycyl-lysine vasopressin) controls acute bleeding oesophageal varices. A double-blind, randomized, placebo-controlled trial. *Scand J Gastroenterol* 1990; **25**: 622–630.

57 Colin R, Giuli N, Czernichow P, Ducrotte P, Lerebours E. Prospective comparison of glypressin, tamponade and their association in the treatment of bleeding esophageal varices. In: Lebrec D, Blei AT (eds), *Vasopressin Analogs and Portal Hypertension*. Paris: John Libbey Eurotext, 1987: 149–153.

58 Fort E, Sautereau D, Silvain C, Ingrand P, Pillegrand B, Beauchant M. A randomized trial of terlipressin plus nitroglycerin vs balloon tamponade in the control of acute variceal hemorrhage. *Hepatology* 1990; **11**: 678–681.

59 Freeman JG, Cobden I, Lishman AH, Record CO. Controlled trial of terlipressin ('glypressin') versus vasopressin in the early treatment of esophageal varices. *Lancet* 1982; **ii**: 66–68.

60 Desaint B, Florent C, Levy VG. A randomized trial of triglycyl-lysine vasopressin versus lysine vasopressin in active cirrhotic variceal hemorrhage. In: Lebrec D, Blei AT (eds), *Vasopressin Analogs and Portal Hypertension*. Paris: John Libbey Eurotext, 1987: 155–157.

61 Lee YF, Tsay YT, Lai KH *et al.* A randomized controlled study of triglycyl-vasopressin and vasopressin plus nitroglycerin in the control of acute esophageal variceal hemorrhage. *Chinese J Gastroenterol* 1988; **5**: 131–138.

62 Chiu WK, Sheen IS, Liaw YF. A controlled study of glypressin versus vasopressin in the control of bleeding from esophageal varices. *J Gastroenterol Hepatol* 1990; **5**: 549–553.

63 D'Amico G, Traina M, Vizzini G *et al.* Terlipressin or vasopressin plus transdermal nitroglycerin in a treatment strategy for digestive bleeding in cirrhosis. A randomized clinical trial. *J Hepatol* 1994; **20**: 206–212.

64 Silvain C, Carpentier S, Sautereau D *et al.* Terlipressin plus transdermal nitroglycerin vs. octreotide in the control of acute bleeding from esophageal varices: a multicenter randomized trial. *Hepatology* 1993; **18**: 61–65.

65 Walker S, Kreichgauer HP, Bode JC. Terlipressin vs somatostatin in bleeding esophageal varices: a controlled double blind study. *Hepatology* 1992; **15**: 1023–1030.

66 Variceal Bleeding Study Group. Double blind comparison of somatostatin infusion vs glypressin injection in the treatment of acute variceal haemorrhage in patients with cirrhosis. *J Hepatol* 1993; 18 (Suppl. 1): S37.

67 Ring EJ, Lake JR, Roberts JP *et al*. Using transjugular intrahepatic portosystemic shunts to control variceal bleeding before liver transplantation. *Ann Intern Med* 1991; 116: 304–309.

68 Le Moine G, Deviere J, Ghysels M *et al*. Transjugular intrahepatic portosystemic stent shunt as a rescue after sclerotherapy failure in variceal bleeding. *Scand J Gastroenterol* 1994; 29 (Suppl. 207): 23–28.

69 Orloff MJ, Chandler JG, Charters AC *et al*. Portacaval shunt as emergency procedure in unselected patients with alcoholic cirrhosis. *Surg Gynecol Obstet* 1975; 141: 59–68.

70 Villeneuve JP, Pomier-Layrargues G, Duguay L *et al*. Emergency portacaval shunt for variceal hemorrhage. *Ann Surg* 1987; 206: 48–55.

71 Pagliaro L, Burroughs AK, Sorensen TIA *et al*. Therapeutic controversies and randomised controlled trials (RCTs): prevention of bleeding and rebleeding in cirrhosis. *Gastroenterology International* 1989; 2: 71–84.

72 Van Stiegmann G. Elastic band ligation of oesophageal varices. In: Bosch J, Groszmann RJ (eds), *Portal Hypertension. Pathophysiology and Treatment*. Oxford: Blackwell Scientific Publications, 1994: 154–163.

73 Merkel C, Morabito A. Adding beta-blockers to sclerotherapy in the prevention of rebleeding: a meta-analysis reassessment. *J Hepatol,* 1994; 21: 918–919.

74 Pagliaro L, D'Amico G, Pasta L *et al*. Portal hypertension in cirrhosis: natural history. In: Bosch J, Groszmann RJ (eds), *Portal Hypertension. Pathophysiology and Treatment*. Oxford: Blackwell Scientific Publications, 1994: 72–92.

75 Blum A. Principles for selection and exclusion (Discussion). In: Tygstrup N, Lachin JM, Juhl E (eds), *The Randomized Clinical Trials and Therapeutic Decisions*. New York, Basel: M Dekker, 1982: 43–57.

76 Markus BH, Dickson ER, Grambsch PM *et al*. Efficacy of liver transplantation in patients with primary biliary cirrhosis. *N Engl J Med* 1989; 320: 1709–1713.

77 Freedman LS, Spiegelhalter D. Application of bayesian statistics to decision making during a clinical trial. *Stat Med,* ;1992; 11: 23–36.

APPENDIX

Textbooks list according to: Mazza JJ. A library of internists VIII. Recommendations from the American College of Physicians. *Ann Intern Med* 1994; 120: 699–720 (modified).

Internal medicine

1 *Cecil Textbook of Medicine*, 16th edn, Wyngarden JB, Smith LH (eds), Philadelphia: WB Saunders 1982.

2 *Cecil Textbook of Medicine*, 17th edn, Wyngarden JB, Smith LH (eds), Philadelphia: WB Saunders 1985.

3 *Cecil Textbook of Medicine*, 18th edn, Wyngarden JB, Smith LH (eds), Philadelphia: WB Saunders 1988.

4 *Cecil Textbook of Medicine*, 19th edn, Wyngarden JB, Smith LH (eds), Philadelphia: WB Saunders 1992.

5 *Conn's Therapy*, Rakel RE (ed.), Philadelphia: WB Saunders 1982.

6 *Conn's Therapy*, Rakel RE (ed.), Philadelphia: WB Saunders 1985.

7 *Conn's Therapy*, Rakel RE (ed.), Philadelphia: WB Saunders 1988.

8 *Conn's Therapy*, Rakel RE (ed.), Philadelphia: WB Saunders 1990.

9 *Conn's Therapy*, Rakel RE (ed.), Philadelphia: WB Saunders 1993.

10 *Conn's Therapy*, Rakel RE (ed.), Philadelphia: WB Saunders 1995.

11 *Current Critical Care Diagnosis and Treatment*, 1st edn, Bongard FS, Sue DY (eds), Norwalk, Connecticut: Large Medical Book 1994.

12 *Current Medical Diagnosis and Treatment*, 2nd edn, Tierney LM, McPhee SJ, Papadakis M (eds), Norwalk, Connecticut: Appleton & Lange 1992.

13 *Current Medical Diagnosis and Treatment*, 3rd edn, Tierney LM, McPhee SJ, Papadakis M (eds), Norwalk, Connecticut: Appleton & Lange 1995.

14 *Harrison's Principles of Internal Medicine*, 11th edn, Isselbacher KJ, Braunwald E, Martin JB, Fauci AS, Kasper DL (eds), New York: McGraw-Hill 1987.

15 *Harrison's Principles of Internal Medicine*, 12th edn, Isselbacher KJ, Braunwald E, Martin JB, Fauci AS, Wilson JD, Kasper DL (eds), New York: McGraw-Hill 1991.

16 *Harrison's Principles of Internal Medicine*, 13th edn, Isselbacher KJ, Braunwald, E, Martin JB, Fauci AS, Wilson, JD, Kasper DL (eds), New York: McGraw-Hill 1994.

17 *Intensive Care Medicine*, 2nd edn, Rippe JM, Irvin RS, Alpert J, Fink MP (eds), Boston: Little, Brown 1991.

18 *Internal Medicine*, 2nd edn, Stein JH (ed.), St Louis: Mosby 1987.

19 *Internal Medicine*, 3rd edn, Stein JH (ed.), St Louis: Mosby 1990.

20 *Internal Medicine*, 4th edn, Stein JH (ed.), St Louis: Mosby 1994.

21 *Manual of Medical Therapeutics*, 26th edn, Woodley W, Whelan A (eds), Boston: Little, Brown 1989.

22 *Manual of Medical Therapeutics*, 27th edn, Woodley M, Whelan A (eds), Boston: Little, Brown 1992.

23 *Oxford Textbook of Medicine*, 1st edn, Weatherall DJ, Ledingham JGG, Warrell DA (eds), Oxford: Oxford University Press 1983.

24 *Oxford Textbook of Medicine*, 2nd edn, Weatherall DJ, Ledingham JGG, Warrell DA (eds), Oxford: Oxford University Press 1987.

25 *Scientific American Medicine*, Rubistein E, Federman DD (eds), New York: *Scientific American* 1995.

26 *Textbook of Internal Medicine*, 1st edn, Kelley W (ed.), Philadelphia: JB Lippincott 1989.

27 *Textbook of Internal Medicine*, 2nd edn, Kelley W (ed.), Philadelphia: JB Lippincott 1992.

Gastroenterology

28 *Bockus Gastroenterology*, 5th edn, Haubrich WS, Schaffner F, Berk P (eds), Philadelphia: WB Saunders 1995.

29 *Clinical Gastroenterology*, 4th edn, Spiro HM (ed.), New York: McGraw-Hill 1993.

30 *Diseases of the Liver*, 5th edn, Schiff L, Schiff ER (eds), Philadelphia: JB Lippincott 1982.

31 *Diseases of the Liver*, 6th edn, Schiff L, Schiff ER (eds), Philadelphia: JB Lippincott 1987.

32 *Diseases of the Liver*, 7th edn, Schiff L, Schiff ER (eds), Philadelphia: JB Lippincott 1993.

33 *Diseases of the Liver and Biliary System*, 6th edn, Sherlock S, Dooley J (eds), Oxford: Blackwell Scientific Publications 1981.
34 *Diseases of the Liver and Biliary System*, 7th edn, Sherlock S, Dooley J (eds), Oxford: Blackwell Scientific Publications 1985.
35 *Diseases of the Liver and Biliary System*, 8th edn, Sherlock S, Dooley J (eds), Oxford: Blackwell Scientific Publications 1989.
36 *Diseases of the Liver and Biliary System*, 9th edn, Sherlock S, Dooley J (eds), Oxford: Blackwell Scientific Publications 1993.
37 *Gastrointestinal Disease: Pathophysiology, Diagnosis, and Management*, 3rd edn, Sleisenger MH, Fordtran JS (eds), Philadelphia: WB Saunders 1983.
38 *Gastrointestinal Disease: Pathophysiology, Diagnosis and Management*, 4th edn, Sleisenger MH, Fordtran JS (eds), Philadelphia: WB Saunders 1989.
40 *Hepatology. A Textbook of Liver Disease*, 2nd edn, Zakim, D, Boyer TD (eds), Philadelphia: WB Saunders 1990.
41 *Oxford Textbook of Clinical Hepatology*, 1st edn, McIntyre N, Benhamou JP, Bircher J, Rizzetto M, Rodes J (eds), Oxford: Oxford University Press 1991.
42 *Textbook of Gastroenterology*, Yamada T, Alpers DH, Owjang C, Powell DW, Silverstein F (eds), Philadelphia: JB Lippincott 1991.

Trials in Portal Hypertension: Valid Meta-analyses and Valid Randomized Clinical Trials

Ulrik Becker, Andrew K. Burroughs, Paul Calés, Christian Gluud, Alessandro Liberati, Alberto Morabito and Fabio Tiné

SUMMARY

This chapter deals with several topics: (i) a new international collaboration – the Cochrane Collaboration – which will facilitate the performance of valid meta-analysis in the field of portal hypertension as in other fields of medicine; (ii) aspects of design of clinical trials; (iii) clinical aspects of randomized clinical trials (RCTs); (iv) statistical aspects of meta-analyses of RCTs; (v) areas where new meta-analyses and new RCTs of treatment of portal hypertension are most needed; and (vi) the possibility to form a Cochrane Collaborate Review Group in portal hypertension.

More than 13 000 patients have been included in more than 190 RCTs on the treatment of variceal bleeding and primary and secondary prophylaxis of variceal bleeding. It is recommended that:

1 the possibilities of the Cochrane Collaboration should be used by the formation of a Systematic Review Group dealing with the treatment of portal hypertension;

2 specific clinical questions should be asked and answers sought through the performance of valid meta-analyses;

3 more uniform protocols should be used in both small and larger RCTs in order to facilitate meta-analysis based on consensus definitions of end points;

4 international consensus should form the basis for the performance of such meta-analyses on a cumulative basis, i.e. a new meta-analysis after each new RCT;

5 meta-analyses should explore the role of heterogeneity;

6 both dichotomous end-points (failure vs. success) and time-dependent responses (survival curves) have to be considered;

7 analyses based on individual data will enable prognostic and therapeutic factors to be evaluated;

8 a number of new RCTs have to be undertaken in both emergency haemostatic treatment and primary and secondary prevention of bleeding caused by portal hypertension;

9   larger RCTs have to be performed in order to obtain more valid results;
10   all RCTs should register centrally at inception or approval;
11   RCTs should include data on quality-of-life and health economics; and
12   RCTs should use structured reporting.

INTRODUCTION

Portal hypertension – most often caused by liver cirrhosis in industrial nations – may, among other consequences, lead to oesophageal varices, gastric varices and portal hypertensive gastropathy. Variceal bleeding has dramatic consequences for the patients and for their physicians as well. In spite of the fact that more than 190 RCTs have been performed to examine the effect of therapies for variceal bleeding, prevention of variceal bleeding and prevention of recurrent bleeding, a number of questions are still unanswered. There are many causes of this.

1   The design and conduct of valid RCTs are difficult [1].

2   It should be realized that one is most often dealing with the treatment of a consequence (bleeding) of a complication (portal hypertension) of an underlying liver disease. Therefore, the prognosis of these patients are heavily influenced by the severity of the underlying liver disease [1] as well as the aetiology of the liver disease (e.g. alcohol) [2]. A number of prognostic factors for variceal bleeding and mortality such as the size and appearance of varices [1], elevation of portal pressure [3], poor nutritional status and short central circulation time [4] may all be relevant.

3   More than 13 000 patients have been enrolled in the more than 190 RCTs that have been published [5,6]. On average this leaves less than 100 patients per trial (or less than 50 patients per treatment arm per trial). So many small trials leave us with the problem of false-negative as well as false-positive trials [7].

There are two solutions to the latter problem. One is to combine the results of the trial through meta-analyses. However, there are a number of aspects that should be taken into account when performing a meta-analysis, including whether all existent and/or relevant RCTs are available for inclusion, the clinical similarity of RCTs making them comparable (entry criteria, treatment, outcome variables, etc.), and the statistical methods, etc. The other effective solution to the problem is only to perform larger RCTs with sufficient power.

Progress in this field can be obtained through different strategies: introduction of new treatment modalities, improvement of available treatment modalities, refinement of indications (i.e. identifying subgroups of patients for whom the treatment is beneficial, without effect, or even harmful), and finally the combination of these modalities [8].

This chapter deals with several topics: (i) a new international collaboration – the Cochrane Collaboration – which will facilitate the performance of valid meta-analysis in the field of portal hypertension as in other fields of medicine; (ii) aspects of design of clinical trials; (iii) clinical aspects of RCTs; (iv) statistical aspects of meta-analyses of RCTs; (v) areas where new meta-analyses and new RCTs of treatment of portal hypertension are most needed; and (vi) the possibility to form a Cochrane Collaborative Review Group in portal hypertension.

THE COCHRANE COLLABORATION

The Cochrane Collaboration is a 2-year-old international research organization [9]. From small beginnings in September 1992 its membership has grown to over 1000 people. It now has eight collaborating centres around the world and 12 registered international review groups dealing with approximately 30 clinical areas. Despite these signs of success, many who could benefit from the collaboration's work, or contribute to it, remain unaware or unsure of its purpose.

Named after the British epidemiologist Archie Cochrane, the Collaboration was set up to evaluate the available evidence from RCTs. Its underlying assumption is that health care interventions will be more effective if they are based on complete and up-to-date evidence instead of out-of-date research, anecdote and conjecture. Its eventual goals are to create a register of all completed and continuing RCTs; to combine the results of trials that meet set standards of quality; to produce regularly updated systematic reviews of meta-analyses; and to make these reviews widely available in journals, on CD-ROM, and eventually on-line through the Internet.

With sophisticated computerized databases such as MEDLINE, finding all RCTs should be a simple matter. However, research has found that about half the 40 000 RCTs published since 1985 are not retrievable by expert MEDLINE searchers. These findings explain why the collaboration places such importance on searching journals by hand. Researchers and some journal editors are volunteering to hand-search journals back to 1948, the year that the *British Medical Journal* published the landmark RCT of streptomycin [10].

Even more taxing than non-indexed trials is the problem of finding trials performed but never published. Despite assumptions that journal editors are biased against publishing negative results, studies have shown that it is largely authors who do the censoring by deciding not to submit them. In addition, we do not know how many trials sponsored by the pharmaceutical and other industries remain unpublished. The marketing advantage in withholding research findings is obvious, but so too are the ethical and opportunity costs in terms of patients, time and money.

Background of the Cochrane Collaboration

Although undertaking high-quality reviews of the effectiveness of clinical interventions has attracted substantial interest, ensuring that clinical practice reflects the available evidence has been relatively neglected. Resources for health services are inevitably limited, and effective practice should be promoted for the benefit of patients. It is the intention of the Cochrane Collaboration to begin to redress the imbalance between evidence of clinical effectiveness and the effectiveness of methods for promoting evidence-based practice, through the systematic location and synthesis of relevant research findings.

Systematic reviews use rigorous methods to locate and synthesize research relevant to clinical decisions. In other words, they attempt to incorporate the same degree of methodological rigour which is expected of primary research. Unfortunately, most literature reviews published in medical journals, whose aims are to summarize the state of knowledge and to influence practice, fail to apply scientific methods of locating and synthesizing all the relevant available evidence. This leads to advice on practice which may not reflect accurately the findings of primary research and, perhaps more obviously, to publishing contradictory guidelines which may perplex clinicians attempting to provide the best available care.

Systematic reviews of clinical interventions are time consuming and locating primary research studies and including them or combining them into reviews may entail considerable efforts among many researchers internationally. For example, the recent antiplatelet trialist collaborative overviews entailed gathering original patient data on 130 000 patients included in over 300 RCTs. However, they are very necessary, as only through systematically reviewing and updating reviews can evidence on clinical effectiveness be made available. Antman et al. [11], comparing the available evidence of the effectiveness of thrombolysis with the recommendations given by experts using non-systematic methods for literature review in textbooks and review articles, found a 13-year delay between convincing evidence becoming available and its incorporation into even half of the recommendations made. Rigour in undertaking research or systematic reviews does not necessarily result in important findings being incorporated into routine practice. For example, despite publication in the *Lancet* in 1988 of a very large pragmatic randomized trial which clearly showed substantial benefit for thrombolysis in treating acute myocardial infarction, a recent study in the UK suggested that only around 20–50% of patients likely to benefit received this treatment during the study period [12].

THE STRUCTURE OF THE COCHRANE COLLABORATION

Although the Cochrane Collaboration is still at an early stage of its development, its basic structure and methods of working have been established. Each reviewer is a member of a collaborative review group, which consists of individuals sharing an interest in a particular topic (e.g. stroke). Collaborative review groups have often grown out of an *ad hoc* meeting of people, who have recognized that they share an interest in preparing and maintaining systematic reviews of RCTs relevant to a particular problem; but review groups have also emerged in other ways.

Even though in the area of gastroenterology several systematic reviews have been reported in the literature on different topics such as the treatment of oesophageal varices, there is not yet any registered collaborative review group in operation.

Once registered, members of the review group seek funding and other support for their activities from whichever sources they consider appropriate. Each collaborative review group is coordinated by an editorial team. The editorial team is responsible for assembling an edited module of the reviews prepared by members of the review group for incorporation in and then dissemination through the *Cochrane Database of Systematic Reviews*. The first issue of the database was released in May 1995 and contained 50 systematic reviews in areas such as stroke, parasitic diseases, schizophrenia, pregnancy and childbirth.

In addition, the team selects reviews contained in the main database for compilation in one or more specialized databases.

The characteristics and activities of a particular collaborative review group – the Cochrane Pregnancy and Childbirth Group – may help to illustrate how these principles work in practice. The group comprises about 30 reviewers and an editorial team of six people. Collectively, the group is currently responsible for maintaining about 600 systematic reviews of RCTs, and for dealing with between 200 and 300 new reports of trials every year. The group includes reviewers in Australia, Canada, Ireland, The Netherlands, South Africa, the UK and Zimbabwe. Each of these reviewers is responsible for obtaining the resources (particularly their time) needed to prepare and maintain the reviews that fall within their respective areas of expertise.

Although most collaborative review groups focus on health problems (e.g. breast cancer) the Collaboration addresses other dimensions of interest through field coordination. A 'field' may refer to a category of health service users (e.g. children), a group of health professionals (e.g. intensivists), a setting for health care (such as less developed countries) or a class of interventions (like physical therapies). People coordinating activities across a field do so by searching specialist sources for relevant studies (e.g. surgical journals), then facilitating the subsequent evolution of more focused, problem-based collaborative review groups; by helping to ensure that priorities and perspectives in the field of interest (e.g. care of the elderly) are reflected in the work of collaborative review groups; and by compiling specialized databases to serve the specific needs of people in the field concerned (e.g. nursing) using all relevant reviews, regardless of the module through which they were contributed to the *Cochrane Database of Systematic Reviews.*

The work of collaborative review groups and field coordination is facilitated in a variety of ways by the work of Cochrane Centres. The characteristics of each Cochrane Centre reflect the interests of the individuals associated with it and the resources made available to them; but the centres share a responsibility for helping to coordinate and support the other elements of the Cochrane Collaboration, and for exploring ways in which the Collaboration can be developed.

The shared responsibilities of the Cochrane Centres include:

1   maintaining a register of people contributing to the Cochrane Collaboration, with information about their individual responsibilities;

2   maintaining a register of published reports of systematic reviews of the effects of health care, so that the Collaboration can build on existing achievements;

3   helping to establish collaborative groups by fostering international collaboration among people with similar interests, participating in exploratory discussions and meetings, helping to organize workshops and in other ways facilitating collaboration;

4   coordinating the Collaboration's contributions to the creation and maintenance of an international register of completed and ongoing RCTs, thus facilitating the first phase of data collection for reviewers;

5   preparing and developing protocols to systematize the preparation of systematic reviews;

6   promoting and undertaking research to improve the quality of systematic reviews;

7   exploring ways of helping the public, health service providers and purchasers, policy makers and the press to make full use of Cochrane reviews; and

8   organizing workshops, seminars, and colloquia to support and guide the development of the Cochrane Collaboration.

META-ANALYSES

Meta-analysis is a key element of the first step of a general 'explicit' process leading to decision on health care interventions [13], a step in which all the evidence on a certain treatment or technology is synthesized to estimate a relevant piece of information on which the decision will be based. This step, while relatively straightforward for some interventions, can be rather complex and not lacking in subjective judgments for others. In a second step of the same process a series of value judgements are used in which such information is weighted (e.g. with respect to harm, available resources and patient's preferences) and the option expected to have the most desirable outcome is chosen, in order to set up policies [14] or to make individual decisions [15]. Better decision-orientated information from RCTs needs to be collected to strengthen the link between these steps [16].

Requirements for meta-analyses

The purpose of meta-analysis is to perform a statistical analysis of a collection of individual studies in order to integrate the results and not merely to review the literature of the field in question [17]. Therefore a meta-analysis is more than a subjective summarizing of research data and requires careful development of a protocol of methods to be used. *Post hoc* decisions should be avoided. A carefully planned and performed meta-analysis is a time-consuming effort and should include the following main elements.

Criteria for considering trials for review

These criteria should describe the types of patients as well as types of interventions and outcomes of interest.

Search strategy and selection of trials [17,18]

The identification of trials will typically include searches in international databases of RCTs (databases of the Cochrane Collaboration, the MED-LINE database). Moreover, the identification of trials will include checking reference lists to identify additional trials and *Science Citation Index* or other bibliographic databases to ensure a complete retrieval of trials. Additional ways to obtain RCTs include writing to the investigators of previous trials and joining conferences. When all potential trials have been identified, trials are selected for review according to predefined criteria, ideally by reviewers who are blind to the journal, authors, institution and results of the trials in question. Disagreements about inclusion of a trial should be solved by consensus.

Statistical and other methods used [17,19]

The method of summarizing results across the different trials should be decided, i.e. which measure of summarization is appropriate (odds ratio, relative risk, number needed to treat, etc.), how should the trials be weighted in the analysis (size, number of events, quality). The reviewers should also decide whether a 'fixed-effect' model or a 'random-effect' model should be applied. Furthermore, a strategy for subgroups analyses should be decided before the meta-analysis when possible in order to avoid *post hoc* analyses which are generally difficult to interpret. A test of heterogeneity should always be incorporated in the analyses.

Quality assessment of the included trials [17,20]

A quality assessment is already included in the selection procedure of trials, but the quality of included trials should be assessed using well-defined criteria – preferably by reviewers blind to the journal, authors, institution and results of the trials in question. Many scoring systems have been developed and probably the most important criteria for assessing the quality of RCTs are methods of randomization, handling of withdrawals and use of blinding of those assessing outcomes [20]. This quality assessment may be used to explain differences in results between trials, in sensitivity analyses and as weights in the summarization of results.

Discussion of results including implications and sources of heterogeneity [17,19,20]

As a main objective of a meta-analysis it should include a discussion of the practical implications and limitations of the obtained results in relation to the present knowledge in the field in question. An important part is a thorough discussion of sources of heterogeneity in the meta-analysis supplemented by subgroup analyses, although these must be interpreted with great caution. This type of discussion, however, is extremely important in generating new hypotheses for future research and meta-analysis.

DESIGN ASPECTS OF THE METHODOLOGICAL REQUIREMENTS OF TRIALS TO FACILITATE META-ANALYSES IN PORTAL HYPERTENSION

The inclusion of all available evidence and the quantitative nature of the method did create among clinicians expectations of objectivity, generalizability and precision with respect to the pooled estimate resulting from meta-analysis. Firm conclusions, however, may not be the rule. Different quality and clinical heterogeneity of trials may flaw comparability among aggregate studies in a way that cannot be reliably accounted for in present

statistical models [21,22]. In the field of portal hypertension, R CTs of prophylactic sclerotherapy do exemplify the issue [23]. So, there is a risk that the
quantitative answer to the broad question about the extent to which a certain
treatment generally influences a certain outcome in the entire body of
available data – although appropriate at a general level of health care policy
decisions – could result in a clinically inadequate input to the real, explicit
process of decision making.

Being dependent on R CTs, meta-analysis depends on the specific pro-
pensity of design of R CTs to bias. An improvement in utilization and quality
of future trials through identification of inadequacies and encouragement of
their resolution is a desirable, as well as expected, scientific feedback of meta-
analysis [24]. A consensus on methodological requirements for design,
conduct and analysis of individual trials in portal hypertension was reached
at the Baveno I workshop [1]. Among the selected requirements, the issues of
double blindness, standard treatment of controls and sample size calculation
deserve some comment.

When possible, while remaining compatible with optimal care, patients,
investigators and/or evaluators must be kept unaware of the treatment to
eliminate bias in ancillary care, patient response and physician evaluation.
Although blinding is least important when the trial focuses on a hard end-
point such as death, in all cases in which the end-point depends on a jud-
gement (such as in determining causes of death or of bleeding or in assessing
failure to control bleeding) blinding is necessary. If blinding of patients and
investigators is difficult because of side effects or therapy itself (as in surgical
or endoscopic-mediated treatments), it would at least be important to assure
the blinding of the outcome assessor, who is making one important end-point
determination. Among the six aspects of blinding of R CTs [25], only the lack
of adequate allocation concealment (up to the point of assignment) has been
associated empirically with bias [20]. As a matter of fact, quality of trials is
judged by the reported method of randomization in the most used scoring
methods. Randomization should be performed in the pharmacy for drugs,
whereas for therapies delivered unblind such as surgery or sclerotherapy,
central telephone randomization or at least sealed opaque envelopes should
be used. The use of invasive procedures in order to obtain blinding of patients
(sham endoscopy) seems to be ethically questionable.

Placebo should be used only in investigating conditions for which there is
no known treatment of proven efficacy [26]. Based on available evidence and
published meta-analyses, the majority of patients are presently treated with
drugs for prophylaxis of first bleeding, whereas surgery or sclerotherapy or
drugs as well are the standard first-line treatments for prevention of
rebleeding. It should be noted that the more bleeding events are reduced as a
result of therapy, the more risk and cost of each intervention is increased as

well (moving from drugs to sclerotherapy and finally to surgery). All interventions are associated with some fraction of non-compliant patients due to different perspectives of individual patients in taking a daily medication, undergoing repeated endoscopies or in considering the trade-off between a short-term risk of operative mortality and a long-term risk of impaired mental function in order to avoid bleeding. So, 'pragmatic' trials, aimed at effectiveness and decision, should be planned in large samples in order to get broad representativeness with respect to decision if the trial results are to be extrapolated [27].

Calculation of sample size is an essential part of design of trials expected to produce conclusive results, which cannot be based on unrealistic estimates of therapeutic effect. Availability of meta-analysis does not justify the planning of inadequately sized RCTs based on the perspective of pooling the same trials to get *a posteriori* power. On the other hand, sample size calculation will always require taking into consideration pragmatic factors such as availability of personnel, funds and participants. Due to standard treatments, it makes no sense to base the sizing of future studies on the assumptions that each treatment is equally effective. Expected rates of bleeding and rebleeding in untreated patients need to be corrected by factors reflecting risk differences or odds reduction taken from individual RCTs or meta-analysis, and realistic minimal clinically relevant differences (which would lead one therapy to be preferred over the standard by considering factors such as severity of disease and cost of therapy) need to be set down. As a result, based on present knowledge, the number of patients required for assessment of effectiveness of new treatments is increased at an order of magnitude which will require the planning of multicenter RCTs and the meta-analysis of such RCTs.

In order to achieve better comparability among trials and clinically meaningful information from meta-analysis, central design issues are:
1 clear identification of a refined question (not too broad) for meta-analysis, specifying the population, intervention and outcomes of interest;
2 *a priori* specification of hypothesis-testing subgroup analyses;
3 agreement among investigators of potentially combinable trials on obtaining the same main data on target patients, treatments and key outcomes, in order to make prospective meta-analysis of high-quality studies a feasible goal;
4 extraction of individual data when those published do not answer questions about intention-to-treat analysis, time-related end-points, subgroups or dose–response relationships; and
5 careful meta-analysis of individual patient's data, aimed to properly account for assumptions on treatment effect within and between trials and the risk of false-positive errors.

CLINICAL ASPECTS OF METHODOLOGICAL REQUIREMENTS OF TRIALS TO FACILITATE META-ANALYSIS

It is axiomatic that good clinical trials are the essential building blocks and cement of a valid meta-analysis. Thus, great emphasis must be placed on the design of the individual clinical trial. The best advice and instruction for this is to be found in Pocock's excellent book [7].

However, before the design of a clinical trial, the purpose or question to be answered must be clearly defined. It should reflect an unanswered or unclear area of clinical practice, such as aspects of management of portal hypertension. It is not ethical to perform a study whose results cannot add to the body of clinical knowledge, because the results of previous studies have already been accepted as best clinical practice by meta-analytical review, or other structured review. This would be the case, for example, for beta-blockers as primary prophylaxis in unselected cirrhotics with varices, which negate the use of placebo. However, in 1994 a banding ligation trial for primary prophylaxis was published against placebo [28].

Secondly, there is an issue of using a minimum core of clinical variables as patient descriptors (based on their known prognostic value or previous consensus), in order to facilitate meta-analysis on individual patient data and to make it easier to establish if one particular trial is comparable with another. This is important, as individual patient data used in a meta-analysis will give more precise results [29]. Good examples in portal hypertension are Poynard *et al.* [30] and Spina *et al.* [31].

Therefore, there must be consensus regarding the clinical variables that must be reported in each trial. Although, as mentioned these may be based principally on known prognostic variables, e.g. those of the Child–Pugh criteria, they should also include those that allow an easy comparison of patient populations, e.g. aetiology of liver disease and age. However, particularly in acute bleeding there are several other factors which are known to influence the clinical course, such as degree of renal impairment and infection, so that there should be a deliberate policy to 'over-include' descriptive variables in individual clinical trials, which can then be translated into the meta-analyses, or if appropriate excluded after statistical analysis.

For trials of primary prevention the major clinical issue is why the patient was endoscoped in the first place, to be a candidate for a primary prophylaxis trial [32]. It is logical that if patients have been known to have varices for many years but have not bled, their risk of bleeding may be less than a patient presenting with fatigue, and found to have cirrhosis and varices. This aspect may explain the extreme variability in baseline bleeding rates in primary prophylaxis studies [23,32,33]. However, it has not been evaluated, as the data are not presented in individual trials, but it needs to be addressed.

For trials of secondary prevention, the major clinical variable is the time interval from admission (for bleeding) at which the patient is randomized or evaluated for the preventive treatment [34]. As rebleeding risk is highest closest to admission, differences of a few days can lead to large differences in rebleeding, which might be as great as the differences being sought or achieved between different treatments. Again, this aspect has not been evaluated in individual trials because the data are not reported, despite evidence that they influence both rebleeding risk and its evaluation [34]. This issue also impinges on the defining of an acute bleeding episode, in terms of time, as there must be a cut-off before it is considered that prevention of rebleeding starts.

The acute bleeding episode is a distinct clinical entity, and there is likely to be a 'biologically' based time frame which can be recognized as representing it. As early rebleeding is so frequent [34], particularly for variceal bleeding [35], it would seem logical to separate what is meant by the acute bleeding episode from a separate bleeding episode which is to be considered the first in a study of secondary prevention. This risk of early rebleeding is highest in the first 5 days. Given that endoscopic therapy, if used acutely, is usually done again electively at between 5 and 7 days, the duration of the acute bleeding episode could be 5 days. If not 5 days, authors must state what interval they have used.

Given the varying definitions for the duration of an acute bleeding episode and the starting point for the analysis of rebleeding, in the responses by experts to a questionnaire used in Session 2 of the Baveno II workshop, it is likely that published trials for prevention of rebleeding have great variability in the starting point for analysis, and may not be strictly comparable. These time intervals are by nature arbitrary, but this problem emphasizes the need to standardize by consensus the end of the acute bleeding episode and the start of rebleeding prevention.

A separate but important point regarding time intervals is the importance of including in meta-analysis, bleeding and death rates within similar time frames of follow-up. The latter give more precise estimates of treatment effects [30,36].

Thirdly, there is a parallel problem of the definition of clinical outcomes. While death itself is easy to define and death due to variceal bleeding was defined in Baveno I as any death occurring within 6 weeks of an admission for variceal bleeding [1], there was no consensus for failure to control bleeding, nor clinically significant bleeding, nor for rebleeding. The latter was defined by some as any rebleed; by others, only that which was clinically significant (with various definitions), and by others it was dependent on the therapy used.

There was also no consensus on defining failure of measures to prevent rebleeding, definitions of these being very dependent on the type of treatment used. This is perplexing, as what would be the clinical outcome evaluated when two of these treatments are compared? These discrepancies have only become apparent during consensus meetings such as Baveno I and Baveno II. If, therefore, rebleeding in one study is defined differently from another, there must be doubt as to whether the studies are comparable. As an example, in the first long-term sclerotherapy trial [37] the definition of rebleeding was that of rebleeding that needed balloon tamponade. The recent results suggesting that somatostatin and octreotide are as effective as emergency injection sclerotherapy [38] may be due to a more accurate (and perhaps different) definition of failure to control acute bleeding, than had been used previously for studies on emergency sclerotherapy. Perhaps minor early rebleeding was previously discounted as failure of sclerotherapy. This is more plausible than believing sclerotherapy has become less effective in time. These examples show the real problems that exist already in the literature. But the real problem is that authors often do not define what they mean by rebleeding, although this is a major end-point, so that a subgroup analysis within a meta-analysis cannot be done.

Thus, it is not only important to achieve consensus on defining end-points which must be reported and analysed in clinical trials, but also individual trials must clearly state which definitions they may be using and evaluating, in addition to the consensus ones, which it is hoped all will report and evaluate.

Similar problems will arise if there is no consensus on measurements of quality-of-life scores, and hospital costs which are being used increasingly in treatment comparisons.

The issues discussed above are the most important clinical aspects of methodological requirements of trials to facilitate meta-analysis. Unfortunately, despite publication of consensus statements and the growing awareness of meta-analyses, old mistakes keep on being made with new therapies such as TIPSS, in which rebleeding and encephalopathy are seldom defined, and in which the interval from bleeding to randomization is not mentioned.

It is important that authors conform to the consensus criteria, not only to make their studies valuable in the light of other reports, but to provide the bricks and mortar for future treatment decisions for the individual patient based on cumulative meta-analyses of portal hypertension trials.

STATISTICAL ASPECTS OF THE METHODOLOGICAL REQUIREMENTS TO FACILITATE META-ANALYSES

An RCT proposes the comparison between the standard therapy and a new therapy [19,39–42]. The comparison is based on the presence and the size of the effect of therapy (EoT). The EoT is measured as the number of patients that do not experience an adverse end-point if the new therapy provides more benefit than the standard. However, similar studies often do not produce similar results. The first reason for disagreement among study outcomes is the presence of heterogeneity, and the following question has to be answered: which role does heterogeneity play? The answer is that a heterogeneous EoT is always present, due to at least four sources of variability aside from chance:

1   different definitions of EoT (odds ratio, risk difference, relative risk);
2   patient selection criteria and unbalancing of risk factors;
3   data imputable to the study design; and
4   inexplicable though real.

Since the comparison among RCTs is based on the experiment similarity in terms of treatment, population of treated and controls, follow-up period, end-points and their validation criteria, one can expect that well-conducted RCTs have to appear similar and conclude that more surprising is an inexplicable heterogeneity of results due to the presence of: (i) unmatched subgroups; (ii) individual prognostic factors; (iii) poor quality of experiments; (iv) definition and verification of end-points; (v) responses related to the stage of disease; and (vi) treatment regimen interacting with the stage of disease. The most popular index for inexplicable heterogeneity is the quality score (Table 23). However, it is still unclear whether quality scores can be of use in a statistical analysis. Some suggestions foresee that one can weight the component of variance in the Der Simonian random model [39,43]. An example of quality criteria of RCTs from the emergency treatment of bleeding in cirrhosis is shown in Table 23.

Meta-analysis of binary response in randomized clinical trials

The aim of the statistical analysis is to compare the number of **observed events in treated patients** with the number of **expected events in treated patients**.

Let us suppose that K homogeneous RCT studies $i=1,\dots,K$ have been enrolled and that the ith study enrols N_i subjects of whom T_i are treated with new treatment, O_i have experienced the end-point of whom O_{Ti} are recruited in the treated group.

The probability for an enrolled patient to experience one end-point is estimated by the proportion of subjects with that end-point

$$P_{\text{End-point}} = \frac{N_{\text{End-point}}}{N_{\text{End-point}}} = \frac{O_i}{N_i}$$

and the probability of being treated with new treatment is estimated by the proportion of subjects receiving new treatment

Table 23 Quality criteria of randomized clinical trials dealing with the treatment of bleeding in cirrhosis.

Quality criteria	Description or reason for use	Score
Randomization method	Blind randomization (on phone call)	(0–6)
Randomization efficacy	Unpaired main prognostic factors	(0–6)
Blindness in treatment	No treatment interaction if it is known	(0–6)
Interim evaluation (blind)	No exclusion of 'invaluable' patients	(0–6)
Patient compliance	Well-completed therapeutic schedule	(0–6)
Study power	*A priori* calculation of sample size	(0–6)
Exclusion rate 15%	Enrolled at least 85% of patients proposed	(0–6)
Intention to treat	Evaluation of all randomized subjects	(0–6)
Correct response evaluation	Survival curves, log-rank test	(0–6)
Study power *a posteriori*	Distribution of withdrawals	(0–6)
Histology	Confirmation of diagnosis	(0–6)
Reference population	... eligible/ineligible patients	(0–6)
Therapeutic regimen	... doses – times – efficacy	(0–6)
Side effects	... toxicity	(0–6)
Cycles and dosages	Number of reduced doses	(0–6)
End-points	Report of mortality and efficacy	(0–6)
Total	Maximum score	96

$$P_{\text{Treated}} = \frac{N_{\text{Treated}}}{N_{\text{Enrolled}}} = \frac{T_i}{N_i}$$

where the number expected among treated patients follows the mathematical model from a null hypothesis:

$$N_{\text{Expected . End-point}} = N_{\text{Treated}} \times P_{\text{End-point}} = N_{\text{End-point}} \times P_{\text{Treated}}$$

The comparison of **similar with similar** (similar for therapy, stratification characteristics, selection criteria and criteria of evaluation of response) in different trials is based on the hypothesis that the statistical observed number of end-points – expected number of end-points would assume a value < 0 when the treatment effect is favourable. The treatment effect is therefore favourable when $O_{T,i} - E_{Ti} < 0$, even if in a particular RCT this tendency can be reversed by chance, by combining the tendencies of each RCT the real tendency should clearly appear by summing the contribute $O_{T,i} - E_{Ti}$ of every single RCT to obtain the EoT

$$\text{EoT} = \sum_{i=1}^{K}(O_{T,i} - E_{T,i})$$

If the treatment is without any effect the value EoT should differ from 0 only randomly. The variance of EoT is the sum of all the variances

$$\text{var}(\text{EoT}) = \sum_{i=1}^{K} \text{var}(O_{T,i} - E_{T,i})$$

It can be shown mathematically that the odds ratio (OR) in each trial for $i = 1, \ldots, K$ is

$$OR_i = \exp\left[\frac{O_{T,i} - E_{T,i}}{\text{var}(O_{T,i} - E_{T,i})}\right]$$

and the OR for the treatment across the studies is

$$OR_T = \exp\left[\frac{\text{EoT}}{\text{var}(\text{EoT})}\right] = \exp\left[\frac{\sum(O_{T,i} - E_{T,i})}{\sum \text{var}(O_{T,i} - E_{T,i})}\right]$$

The confidence limits of OR can be easily calculated, as the upper and the lower limit:

$$OR_{\text{Upper}} = \exp\left[\frac{\text{EoT}}{\text{var}(\text{EoT})} + \frac{1.96}{\text{se}(\text{EoT})}\right] \text{ and}$$

$$OR_{\text{Lower}} = \exp\left[\frac{\text{EoT}}{\text{var}(\text{EoT})} - \frac{1.96}{\text{se}(\text{EoT})}\right]$$

where $\text{se}(\text{EoT})$ is the standard error of EoT.

The **efficient score** statistic is given by:

$$Z_i = O_{T,i} - \frac{O_i \times T_i}{N_i} = O_{T,i} - E_{T,i}$$

and the Fisher information is given by:

$$V_i = \frac{O_i}{N_i} \times \frac{(N_i - O_i)}{N_i} \times \frac{(N_i - T_i) \times T_i}{(N_i - 1)}$$

It can be shown that asymptotically the statistic Z_i has a Gauss distribution with variance V_i. From this property, one derives the significance test and the confidence limits for the EoT.

The validity of estimate $\Sigma(O-E)$ as EoT requires implicitly the availability of all the data of all the RCTs and the absence of any systematic error due to the lack of negative or unpromising results due to loss of patients to follow-up. The advantages of meta-analysis consist of the fact that it is not necessary to compare patients directly in different RCTs and that it is not necessary for the true value of EoT to be the same in all the RCTs.

Meta-analysis of survival data in randomized clinical trials

Let us suppose that every study records the time between the random assignment to a therapy and the appearance of the defined event. In the study *i*th, the events occur at m[*i*] different times $t_{(1,i)}, \ldots, t_{(m[i],i)}$. At each of these times no more than one event can occur. However, because of numeric rounding or because of the protocol of RCT imposing scheduled follow-up time, it can occur that more than one event is measured in the same time interval.

The events $O_{j,i}$ occur at the times $t_{j,i}$, for, $j = 1, \ldots, m[i]$, and the total number of events is: $e_i = o_1 + \ldots + o_{m[i],i}$. Some **survival times** can be censored on the right, thereafter it is necessary to record them separately for each of *j* times in correspondence of which $r_{(j,i)}$ patients have survival times $\geq t_{(j,i)}$, that is the **risk set** at the times $t_{(j,i)}$.

Models and data for *i*th RCT are shown in Table 24. The risk functions for <E-group> receiving the experimental treatment and for <C-group> receiving the standard treatment, are respectively: $^h E, i^{(t)}$ and $^h C, i^{(t)}$. On the hypothesis of **proportional risk** EoT is equal to a constant estimated by the logarithm of the ratio of the two risk functions

$$EoT = -log\{h_{E,i}(t)/h_{C,i}(t)\}, \text{ for } t > 0$$

This formula is also the difference of minus the logarithmic functions of log **survivors**,

$$EoT = -log(-log[S_{E,i}(t)]) + log(-log[S_{C,i}(t)]), \text{ for each } t_j > 0.$$

The statistical justification of the estimate of the confidence limits of the odds ratio is given by the **efficient score statistics** asymptotically normally distributed

$$Z_i = e_{Ci} - \sum_{j=1}^{m(i)} \frac{o_{j,i} r_{jC,i}}{r_{j,i}}$$

and the Fisher information

Table 24 Survival data from RCT *i*th.

Model	Treated	Controls	Overall
Hazard function	$h_E(t)$	$h_C(t)$	$h(t)$
Surviving fraction	$S_E(t)$	$S_C(t)$	$S(t)$
No. of events	e_E	e_C	$e(t)$

Observed events at time *T* and after survival time *T*.

$T =$				$T \geqslant$			
t_1	$O_{E,1}$	$O_{C,1}$	O_1	t_1	$r_{E,1}$	$r_{C,1}$	r_1
....				....			
$t_{m[i]}$	$O_{E,m[i]}$	$O_{C,m[i]}$	$O_{m[i]}$	$t_{m[i]}$	$r_{E,m[i]}$	$r_{C,m[i]}$	$r_{m[i]}$

$$V_i = \sum_{j=1}^{m(i)} \frac{o_{j,i} r_{jC,i} (r_{j,i} - o_{j,i}) r_{jE,i}}{(r_{j,i} - 1) r_{j,i}^2}$$

Moreover, Z_i coincides with the log-rank statistic and V_i with the variance of the null hypothesis $H_0 : O_T - E_T = 0$ with variance V_T as well [44]. The reference model is the **proportional hazard stratified**, with proportionality among centres not necessarily required. The value of statistic X^2 for log-rank test can be derived:

$$X^2 \approx \frac{Z^2}{V_T}$$

Moreover, e_i the total number of events of each study can be estimated since:

$$V_i \approx \frac{1}{4} e_i$$

From this information, V_i and Z_i can be roughly estimated. The statistics are presented in *The Design and Analysis of Sequential Clinical Trials* [45].

Alternatively, the Cox survival model [46] could have been adjusted and the regression coefficients could have been referred jointly with their standard errors. Such coefficients are the estimates $\overline{\text{EoT}}_i$ of the true EoT_i and approximately hold that:

$$Z_i = \overline{\text{EoT}}_i \cdot \text{se}(\overline{\text{EoT}}_i)^{-2} , \quad V_i = \text{se}(\overline{\text{EoT}}_i)^{-2}$$

One must be careful in using such derived estimates. The authors of published papers might have used different rules and terminology from the ones used in these pages and in this way the identification of approximate statistics becomes difficult. Finally, the correspondence with sure and valid values must follow an accurate calculation of these statistics.

PUBLISHED META-ANALYSIS IN PORTAL HYPERTENSION

Based among others on a MEDLINE search, a total of 23 meta-analyses on treatment of portal hypertension have been identified [6,23,30,31, 33,36,38,47–62]. All meta-analyses have dealt with treatment of oesophageal or gastric varices. No meta-analyses have been published on treatment of portal hypertensive gastropathy. In fact, very few RCTs on treatment and primary and secondary prophylaxis of variceal bleeding have taken portal hypertensive gastropathy into consideration.

Haemostatic treatment

Five meta-analyses have dealt with haemostatic control of bleeding varices. Three meta-analyses on the effect of somatostatin and octreotide have been published as letters or are in press [38,57,61]. One comprehensive meta-analysis on different treatment modalities has been published as an abstract [53] and one dealing with almost the same studies as the latter has been published as a proceeding from a symposium [6]. It is puzzling that so few meta-analyses have been performed considering the vast number of papers that have been published since the 1950s dealing with pharmacological and other treatment approaches.

The key end-point is bleeding control. At the Baveno I workshop no consensus could be reached on the definition of clinically significant bleeding or definition of duration of acute bleeding episodes and evaluation parameters to monitor bleeding control [1]. Further, patients without active bleeding at the time of endoscopy but with endoscopically proven varices pose a diagnostic problem. These and other problems are reflections of the heterogeneity among trials. The different trials vary greatly in success rates in control groups, inclusion criteria and referral pattern, and in many studies the details reported are so inadequate that meta-analysis based on published information is impossible or at best difficult to interpret [6,53]. It is interesting to note that balloon tamponade has never been tested against placebo.

The validity of these results remain to be demonstrated in additional meta-analyses (and RCTs) evaluating each treatment separately. In fact, a meta-analysis comparing somatostatin with placebo was unable to demonstrate any significant effect on control of bleeding or mortality [61]. However, somatostatin or octreotide did not differ significantly from sclerotherapy in obtaining bleeding control [39].

Other treatment comparisons do not demonstrate significant advantages regarding bleeding control or survival [6]. Irrespective of the treatment used, the observed effects have all been small or marginal.

Primary prophylaxis

Twelve meta-analyses have been published on primary prophylaxis of variceal bleeding [23,30,33,48–52,54–56,59]. Ten meta-analyses deal with beta-blocker treatment vs. non-active treatment, four with sclerotherapy vs. non-active treatment and one with shunt surgery vs. non-active treatment. No meta-analyses have been published on the comparison of two active treatments.

As pointed out by Pagliaro *et al.* [33], there seems to be great variability in patient selection and technique in the different trials. In order to encompass some of the problems of performing meta-analysis using heterogenous trials Poynard *et al.* [30] published a meta-analysis based on individual patient data from four trials. They could show that the efficacy of beta-blocker treatment was greatest among patients with good compliance, patients without ascites and patients in good condition.

In future meta-analyses it is important to predefine subgroup analysis and/or perform meta-analyses based on individual patient data in order to identify the control for risk factors and imbalances between studies. The predictive value of haemodynamic evaluation on the therapeutic outcome remains to be determined.

Secondary prophylaxis

Fourteen meta-analyses have been published on secondary prophylaxis of variceal bleeding – two as letters [31,33,36,47–52,54,55,58,60,62]. Nine meta-analyses deal with beta-blocker treatment vs. non-active treatment, two with sclerotherapy vs. non-active or conventional treatment, one with shunt surgery vs. non-active treatment, two with sclerotherapy vs. beta-blocker, one with sclerotherapy vs. sclerotherapy + beta-blocker, one with sclerotherapy vs. ligation, one with shunt surgery vs. another type of shunt surgery, and one meta-analysis deals with shunt surgery vs. sclerotherapy.

It is interesting to note that one cumulative meta-analysis has demonstrated that beta-blocker treatment (compared with control or placebo) prevented significantly the risk of rebleeding from varices in 1987 and dying in 1990 in cirrhotic patients [58]. However, 46% of the RCTs comparing beta-blocker with non-active treatment appeared after 1987 [5]. None of these RCTs had a sample size aiming at demonstrating an effect on mortality, but rather on the rebleeding rate.

No meta-analysis has employed individual patient data, and again the main problem with meta-analysis in this field is heterogeneity within and between trials. It is often difficult to take these factors into account because of inadequate reporting. As an example of important risk factors for therapeutic outcome and a potential source of heterogeneity, Møller *et al.* [63] found that patients with disturbed brain and renal function should not receive sclerotherapy.

Quality of meta-analyses

As previously pointed out, a meta-analysis should be performed according to a defined research strategy and that strategy should be described in the published analysis. In order to obtain a general overview of the quality of

Table 25 Evaluation of meta-analyses on portal hypertension treatment. The figures indicate the number of meta-analyses that adequately describe the quality requirements indicated.

Requirements	Haemostatic treatment ($n = 5$)	Primary prophylaxis ($n = 11$)*	Secondary prophylaxis ($n = 12$)*
Search strategy	1	8	3
Selection of trials	1	8	4
Statistical methods	4	10	10
End-point definition			
bleeding control	2	1	1
mortality	2	5	4

* Not all of the published meta-analyses were included.

meta-analyses on portal hypertension treatment, the majority of the identified meta-analyses were screened for their description of certain central quality requirements. As shown in Table 25, a number of meta-analyses did not meet the quality requirements regarding description of search strategy, trial selection, statistical methods and end-point definition.

Recommendations for new meta-analysis in portal hypertension

The number of meta-analyses is increasing in the evaluation of therapies for portal hypertension. The increasing number, using different selection criteria and methods for evaluation, leads to increasing complexity of these therapeutic areas.

Therefore, the following are generally recommended.

1   It is imperative that consensus is reached on relevant end-points.

2   International Cochrane Collaborative Review Groups should be formed. They should review the existing literature according to the guidelines of the Cochrane Collaboration. Forming Cochrane Review Groups is considered an excellent way of performing meta-analyses in a standardized way. They also guarantee the results will be updated as new trials emerge.

3   All therapies should be monitored by cumulative meta-analyses. A new meta-analysis should be performed when additional evidence is published.

4   Subgroup analysis. This should be based on predefined hypotheses, on potential sources of heterogeneity and if possible take prognostic and therapeutic factors into account.

5   Meta-analysis based on individual patient data. Although time-consuming, this is possibly the best way of reducing some of the heterogeneity between and within trials, on the condition that the source of heterogeneity is

known. Furthermore, the analysis of individual patient data allows prognostic and therapeutic factors to be evaluated.

6   Treatment of the acute bleeding episode. Comprehensive meta-analyses on the treatment of the acute bleeding episode should have a high priority, preferably based on analyses of individual patient data.

7   Incorporation of prognostic and therapeutic variables. Analyses based on individual data will enable prognostic and therapeutic factors to be evaluated as, for example, haemodynamic variables, endoscopic appearance, ascites, encephalopathy, renal function, Child criteria, active alcohol abuse, presence of portal hypertensive gastropathy and aetiology of the liver disease.

8   Health economic analyses and complications. Future meta-analyses should also take health economics analyses, side-effects and complications into consideration and not only focus on treatment effect.

INDICATION OF AREAS WHERE NEW TRIALS ARE MOST NEEDED IN THERAPY AND PRIMARY AND SECONDARY PROPHYLAXIS OF PORTAL HYPERTENSION

The study of portal hypertension is a growing field and new RCTs are published every month. This activity reflects the multiplicity of therapeutic methods, of statistical methods and of unanswered questions. For each of the three therapeutic areas on this topic, the following account will first present the background and will conclude with suggestions for therapeutic options. The background relies on the analyses of three types of data: (i) previous consensus meetings [1,64]; (ii) cumulative analyses of published RCTs and their meta-analysis when available; and (iii) promising new therapeutic methods with only a few preliminary reports or without any published RCTs.

Haemostatic treatment

At the Baveno I workshop, consensus could only be achieved on the following statement: 'In every centre a treatment strategy should be defined, with several steps to control the bleeding episode not only for 24 hours, but for a few days (e.g. 5) . . .' [1]. A more detailed strategy was defined in another consensus meeting, but this reflected a national opinion [64]. At the end of 1994, 69 RCTs had been published [65], of which 37 (54%) were published between 1990 and 1994, i.e. after the Baveno I workshop.

The significant new results since Baveno I are the following: (i) the main data concern pharmacological treatment which compares favourably with other methods especially endoscopic treatments; (ii) the combination of endoscopic sclerotherapy with pharmacological treatment seems to improve the efficacy of sclerotherapy for bleeding; and (iii) band ligation seems as effective as sclerotherapy although more difficult in an emergency room. There are no RCTs with TIPS, but uncontrolled trials suggest that TIPS is effective for uncontrolled bleeding (secondary haemostasis).

A novel concept has recently emerged: the pharmacological treatment by a mobile intensive care unit before hospitalization seems to improve primary haemostasis and overall mortality at 6 weeks. There is only a (preliminary) report of one RCT devoted solely to gastric varices.

Recommendations

Randomized clinical trials on haemostatic treatment of acute variceal bleeding should define more powerful predictive factors of continued bleeding and more powerful therapeutic response. Experimental treatments must be tested against treatment options for which there exists evidence of a beneficial effect.

In acute oesophageal variceal bleeding, based on the present knowledge, RCTs could evaluate:
- vasoactive drugs vs. placebo in addition to endoscopic treatment (banding ligation or sclerotherapy);
- comparison of variable vasoactive drug treatment durations (e.g. 2 vs. 5 days) in addition to endoscopic treatment;
- TIPS vs. endoscopic treatment;
- TIPS vs. shunt surgery;
- the sequential combination of different treatment approaches; and
- different forms of sclerosant/adhesive for endoscopic treatment.

In acute gastric variceal bleeding, based on the present knowledge, RCTs could evaluate:
- TIPS vs. endoscopic treatment (tissue adhesive and/or band ligation); and
- vasoactive drugs vs. placebo in addition to endoscopic treatment.

Primary prophylaxis

The following consensus was achieved in the Baveno I workshop: 'All patients with high variceal bleeding risk should receive prophylaxis of first variceal bleeding. At the moment, beta-blockers are the best candidate drugs' [1].

At the end of 1994, 42 RCTs had been published of which 20 (48%) were published between 1990 and 1994 [5]. At present, beta-blockers are the recommended treatment in this situation. However, one RCT suggested that organic nitrates may be an alternative to beta-blockers and one preliminary study has suggested that the combination of beta-blockers + organic nitrates could be more effective than beta-blockers alone for bleeding incidences.

One other preliminary report suggested that endoscopic band ligation could reduce the incidence of first variceal bleeding. Japanese authors have demonstrated that portal non-decompression surgery was effective in preventing variceal bleeding and in improving survival. In one recent RCT, Paquet *et al.* [66] concluded that prophylactic endoscopic sclerotherapy reduces the incidence of first variceal bleeding and can prolong survival if only high-risk patients are selected and the treatment is performed by endoscopic experts. Moreover, a recent meta-analysis has suggested that prophylactic sclerotherapy with polidocanol was effective, particularly in high-risk patients [59].

Recommendations

Randomized clinical trials on primary prevention of variceal bleeding should define more powerful predictive factors associated with first variceal bleeding and more powerful therapeutic response. Experimental treatments must be tested against treatment options for which there exists evidence of a beneficial effect, e.g. beta-blockers in tolerant patients.

Based on the present knowledge, RCTs could evaluate:
- beta-blockers vs. nitrates alone or in combination with beta-blockers;
- beta-blockers vs. long-acting somatostatin analogue alone or in combination with beta-blockers;
- beta-blockers vs. banding ligation alone or in combination with beta-blockers.

Randomized clinical trials could also evaluate therapies directed towards the cause of elevated portal pressure, e.g. antifibrotics. Such preventive measures could be called preprimary prevention. Trials could also be aimed at preventing the occurrence of (large) varices.

Secondary prophylaxis

In the Baveno I workshop no precise strategy could be defined. However, a consensus was achieved on the following guidelines: (i) first choice: no treatment is not justified – endoscopic sclerotherapy or beta-blockers or surgery can be used; (ii) if the first choice of treatment failed, one of the three previous treatments or liver transplantation can all be used; (iii) first choice for prevention of gastric variceal rebleeding – beta-blockers. Surgery and endoscopic sclerotherapy can, however, be used [1].

At the end of 1994, 80 RCTs had been published of which 36 (45%) were published between 1990 and 1994 [5]. Some new information had become available since the Baveno I workshop.

1   Beta-blockers: the most recent meta-analysis (12 RCTs) had shown a

significant decrease in the incidence of rebleeding and overall mortality compared with control patients [58].

2   Sclerotherapy had been compared with other treatments. The results demonstrated the following findings:

(a) a recent meta-analysis of nine RCTs showed that sclerotherapy was more effective in preventing rebleeding than beta-blockers, but there was no significant difference in 2-year survival [36];

(b) a meta-analysis of 10 RCTs showed that, compared with sclerotherapy, band ligation significantly decreased the rate of bleeding and complications but not mortality [62];

(c) another analysis suggested that the combination of beta-blockers + sclerotherapy was more effective than sclerotherapy alone for rebleeding, but there was a significant heterogeneity among the RCTs [60];

(d) sclerotherapy was compared with TIPS in four RCTs. Preliminary results showed that rebleeding was significantly decreased with TIPS, but the death rate was similar.

The analysis of effectiveness of treatments is more difficult in secondary prevention since it is not always possible to distinguish between what is attributable to the effect of haemostatic treatment and to the prevention of rebleeding. For example, it has been suggested that the effects of emergency sclerotherapy were not different from those of elective sclerotherapy.

Recommendations

Again, more powerful predictive factors of recurrent variceal bleeding and therapeutic response must be defined. Moreover, experimental treatments must be tested against treatment options for which there exists evidence of a beneficial effect.

It is now necessary to test the additive effects of treatments especially by using drugs with different action sites [67]. The criteria leading to optimal dosage and association of drugs must be defined. Based on present knowledge, RCTs could evaluate:

• long-acting somatostatin analogue vs. beta-blocker;
• nitrates vs. placebo in addition to beta-blocker;
• banding ligation vs. drug therapy;
• beta-blocker vs. placebo in addition to endoscopic treatment (banding ligation or sclerotherapy);
• TIPS vs. endoscopic treatment (banding ligation or sclerotherapy);
• TIPS vs. partial portocaval shunts; and
• surgical procedures (partial portocaval shunts or extensive devascularisation) vs. endoscopic treatment (banding ligation or sclerotherapy) plus drug therapy.

LARGER RANDOMIZED CLINICAL TRIALS AND CENTRAL TRIAL REGISTRATION

The observations that more than 13 000 patients have been randomized in more than 190 RCTs demonstrate that both patients and physicians are willing to participate in RCTs in this field. In future RCTs, this willingness ought to be translated into larger RCTs having sufficient power. Combining such large RCTs with analyses of quality of life and health economics will facilitate the implementation of the results of clinical research into clinical practice. Further, RCTs should use structured reporting [68] and include data on consensus end-points, even if those chosen by authors are not the same. This will also facilitate meta-analyses.

Any RCT, small or large, should register an inception or approval and at termination of the RCT [69]. Such registers are being planned in the Cochrane Collaboration and may facilitate cooperation and harmonization and reduce duplication.

COCHRANE COLLABORATIVE REVIEWS OF TRIALS IN PORTAL HYPERTENSION

As demonstrated, the number of RCTs and meta-analyses is increasing in the area of therapy of variceal bleeding. Variation in inclusion criteria, the therapeutic options, end-points and methods of performing meta-analysis are making this therapeutic area difficult to overlook.

In order to create consensus in this area, our option is to perform meta-analyses that use the most objective methods to evaluate the results of available RCTs. The Cochrane Collaboration may facilitate this goal. A number of scientists have expressed their interest to participate in Cochrane Collaborative Reviews and more are expected to join. The main objectives for the Cochrane Reviewers should be as follows.

1   Hand-search specialist journals etc. for RCTs (all RCTs, not only RCTs dealing with portal hypertension). Some researchers have already registered. However, there is a huge need for additional researchers that will take on the responsibility to hand-search journals both back in time and on an ongoing basis. They should register at the Baltimore Cochrane Centre [9].

2   Analyse and synthesize these RCTs if possible by means of meta-analyses. At the present time, only preliminary registration has taken place. However, a number of physicians have expressed their keen interest in joining a Collaborative Review Group dealing with portal hypertension.

The Australasian Cochrane Centre is currently responsible for maintaining a directory of people who are either already contributing to the Cochrane Collaboration or who have contacted one of the Cochrane Centres expressing an interest in doing so. The UK Cochrane Centre has assembled a directory of published and some unpublished reports of systematic reviews of RCTs. People considering establishing a new collaborative review group should consult both these resources.

After a group has agreed to form a Collaborative Review Group to undertake ongoing responsibility, for the foreseeable future, the final step is to formalize the existence of the group as part of the Cochrane Collaboration. The group should prepare a report of the group's deliberations and conclusions. The report should be sent to the Director of the nearest Cochrane Centre for comment. An agreed version of the report should then be sent to the Chair of the Collaboration's Steering Group [9].

REFERENCES

1 de Franchis R, Pascal JP, Ancona E *et al.* Definitions, methodology and therapeutic strategies in portal hypertension. A consensus development workshop, Baveno, Lake Maggiore, Italy, April 5–6, 1990. *J Hepatol* 1992; **15**: 256–261.

2 Cristani A, Cioni G, Tincani E, Sardini C, Ventura E. Effect of alcohol abstinence on oesophageal varices and portal hypertensive gastropathy in patients with liver cirrhosis. *Alcologia* 1994; **6**(3): 207–213.

3 Gluud C, Henriksen JH, Nielsen G and the Copenhagen Study Group for Liver Disease. Prognostic indicators in alcoholic cirrhotic men. *Hepatology* 1988; **8**: 222–227.

4 Møller S, Bendtsen F, Christensen E, Henriksen JH. Prognostic variables in patients with cirrhosis and oesophageal varices without prior bleeding. *J Hepatol* 1994; **21**: 940–946.

5 Calès P, Oberti F. Prévention de la rupture des varices oesophagiennes. *Enc Med Chir* 1995; **1**: 7034-D-15.

6 de Franchis R. Treatment of bleeding oesophageal varices: a meta-analysis. *Scand J Gastroenterol* 1994; **29** (Suppl. 207): 29–33.

7 Pocock SJ. *Clinical Trials. A Practical Approach.* Chichester: John Wiley, 1983.

8 Sørensen TIA. Failure of combined efforts: propranolol and sclerotherapy do not add up to the prevention of variceal bleeding. *J Hepatol* 1993; **19**: 197–199.

9 Sackett D, Oxman A (eds), *The Cochrane Collaboration Handbook.* Oxford: The Cochrane Collaboration, 1994.

10 Medical Research Council. Streptomycin treatment of pulmonary tuberculosis. *Br Med J* 1948; **ii**: 769–782.

11 Antman EM, Lau J, Kupelnick B, Mosteller F, Chalmers TC. A comparison of results of meta-analyses of randomized control trials and recommendations of clinical experts. *JAMA* 1992; **268**: 240–248.

12 Ketley D, Woods KL. Impact of clinical trials on clinical practice: example of thrombolysis for acute myocardial infarction. *Lancet* 1993; **344**: 347–348.

13 Eddy DM. *A Manual for Assessing Health Practices and Designing Practice Policies. The Explicit Approach.* American College of Physicians, 1992: 1–126.

14 Bailar JC III, Mosteller F. Medical technology assessment. In: Bailar JC III, Mostellers F (eds), *Medical Uses of Statistics.* Boston, Massachusetts: NEMJ Books, 1992: 393–411.

15 Wong JB, Salem DN, Pauker SG. You're never too old. *N Engl J Med* 1993; **328**: 971–974.

16 Hilden J, Habbema JK. The marriage of clinical trials and clinical decision science. *Stat Med* 1990; **9**: 1243–1257.

17 Dickersin K, Berlin JA. Meta-analysis: State-of-the-Science. *Epidemiol Rev* 1992; **14**: 154–176.

18 Dickersin K, Scherer R, Lefebvre C. Identifying relevant studies for systematic reviews. *Br Med J* 1994; **309**: 1286–1291.

19 Thompson SG. Why sources of heterogeneity in meta-analysis should be investigated. *Br Med J* 1994; **309**: 1351–1355.

20 Schulz KF, Chalmers I, Hayes RJ, Altman DG. Empirical evidence of bias. Dimensions of methodological quality associated with estimates of treatment effects in controlled trials. *JAMA* 1995; **273**: 408–412.

21 Pocock SJ, Hughes MD. Estimation issues in clinical trials and overviews. *Stat Med* 1990; **8**: 657–671.

22 Kassirer J. Clinical trials and meta-analysis. What do they do for us? *N Eng J Med* 1992; **327**: 273–274.

23 Pagliaro L, D'Amico G, Sørensen TIA *et al*. Prevention of first bleeding in cirrhosis. A meta-analysis of randomized trials of nonsurgical treatment. *Ann Int Med* 1992; **117**: 59–70.

24 O'Rourke K, Detsky AS. Meta-analysis in medical research: strong encouragement for higher quality in individual research efforts. *J Clin Epidemiol* 1989; **42**: 1021–1024.

25 Chalmers TC, Berrier J. Randomized control trials, and meta-analysis of the treatment of cirrhosis of the liver. In: Tygstrup N, Orlandi F (eds), *Cirrhosis of the Liver. Methods and Fields of Research*. Amsterdam: Elsevier, 1987: 483–493.

26 Rothman KJ, Michels KB. The continuing unethical use of placebo controls. *N Engl J Med* 1994; **331**: 394–398.

27 Schwartz D, Lellouch J. Explanatory and pragmatic attitudes in therapeutic trials. *J Chron Dis* 1067; **20**: 637–648.

28 Sarin SK, Guptan RC, Jain A. A randomized controlled trial of endoscopic band ligation for primary prophylaxis of variceal bleeding (abstract). *Gastroenterology* 1994; **106**: A975.

29 Steward LA, Parmar MKB. Meta-analysis of the literature or of individual patient data: is there a difference? *Lancet* 1993; **341**: 418–422.

30 Poynard T, Calès P, Pasta L *et al*. Beta-adrenergic-antagonist drugs in the prevention of gastrointestinal bleeding in patients with cirrhosis and esophageal varices. *N Engl J Med* 1991; **324**: 1532–1538.

31 Spina GP, Henderson JM, Rikkers LF *et al*. Distal spleno-renal shunt versus endoscopic sclerotherapy in the prevention of variceal rebleeding. A meta-analysis of 4 randomized clinical trials. *J Hepatol* 1992; **16**: 338–345.

32 Burroughs AK, D'Heygere F, McIntyre N. Pitfalls in prophylactic studies for variceal bleeding. *Hepatology* 1986; **6**: 407–1413.

33 Pagliaro L, Burroughs AK, Sørensen TIA *et al*. Therapeutic controversies and randomized controlled trials (RCT): prevention of bleeding and rebleeding in cirrhosis. *Gastroenterol Int* 1989; **2**: 71–84.

34 Burroughs AK, Mezzanotte G, Philips A, McCormick PA, McIntyre N. Cirrhotics with variceal haemorrhage: the importance of the time interval between admission and the start of analysis for survival and rebleeding rates. *Hepatology* 1989; **9**: 801–807.

35 McCormick PA, Jenkins SA, McIntyre N, Burroughs AK. Why portal hypertensive varices bleed and bleed: a hypothesis. *Gut* 1995; **36**: 100–103.

36 Bernard B, Lebrec D, Mathurin P, Opolon P, Poynard T. Meta-analysis of propranolol

and endoscopic sclerotherapy in the prevention of gastrointestinal rebleeding in patients with cirrhosis (abstract). *Hepatology* 1994; **20**: 106A.

37 Terblanche J, Kahn D, Campbell JAH *et al*. Failure of repeated injection sclerotherapy to improve long-term survival after oesophageal variceal bleeding. *Lancet* 1983; **ii**: 1328–1332.

38 Avgerinos A, Armonis A, Raptis S. Somatostatin or octreotide versus endoscopic sclerotherapy in acute variceal haemorrhage: a meta-analysis study. *J Hepatol* 1995; **22**: 247–251.

39 DerSimonian R, Laird R. Meta-analysis in clinical trials. *Controlled Clinical Trials* 1986; **7**: 177–188.

40 Jones DR. Meta-analysis: weighting the evidence. *Stat Med* 1994; **14**: 137–149.

41 Whitehead A, Whitehead J. A general parametric approach to the meta-analysis of randomised clinical trials. *Stat Med* 1991; **10**: 1665–1677.

42 Whitehead A, Jones NMB. A meta-analysis of clinical trials involving different classification of response into ordered categories. *Stat Med* 1994; **13**: 2503–2515.

43 Berkey CS, Hoaglin D, Mosteller F, Colditz GA. A random-effects regression model for meta-analysis. *Stat Med* 1995;**14**: 395–411.

44 Armitage P, Barry G. *Statistical Methods in Medical Research*. Oxford: Blackwell Scientific Publications, 1993.

45 Whitehead J. *The Design and Analysis of Sequential Clinical Trials*. Chichester: Harwood 1992.

46 Cox DR. Regression models and life tables. *J R Stat Soc B* 1972; **34**: 187–202.

47 Infante-Rivard C, Esnaola S, Villeneuve J-P. Role of endoscopic variceal sclerotherapy in the long-term management of variceal bleeding: a meta-analysis. *Gastroenterology* 1989; **96**: 1087–1092.

48 Lewis JA, Davis JM, Allsopp D, Cameron HA. Beta-blockers in portal hypertension. An overview. *Drugs* 1989; **37** (Suppl. 2): 62–69.

49 Hayes PC, Davis JM, Lewis, Bouchier IAD. Meta-analysis of value of propranolol in prevention of variceal haemorrhage. *Lancet* 1990; **336**: 153–156.

50 Pagliaro L, Burroughs AK, Sørensen TIA. Beta-blockers for preventing variceal bleeding. *Lancet* 1990; **336**: 1001–1002.

51 Lebrec D. Medical treatment of portal hypertension. *Presse Med* 1991; **20**: 750–755.

52 RiccaRosellini S, Miglio F. Beta-blockers for the prevention of variceal haemorrhage in patients with cirrhosis: an updated meta-analysis of randomized controlled trials. *Ital J Gastroenterol* 1991; **23**: 408–415.

53 Burroughs A, Morabito A, de Franchis R, Bosch J, Franco D, Akriviadis E. *Treatment of Acute Oesophageal Variceal Bleeding – A Meta-analytical Study*. Royal Tunbridge Wells: Wells Medical, 1992: 5–7.

54 Dumitrescu DL. Beta-blockers in the prevention of the rupture of oesophageal varices. A meta-analysis. *Med Interna* 1992; **44**: 28–33.

55 Pagliaro L, D'Amico G, Tiné F, Pasta L. Prevention of upper gastrointestinal bleeding from portal hypertension in cirrhosis: rationale for medical treatment. *Dig Dis* 1992; **10** (Suppl. 1): 56–64.

56 Ruiswyk J Van, Byrd JC. Efficacy of prophylactic sclerotherapy for prevention of a first variceal hemorrhage. *Gastroenterology* 1992; **102**: 587–597.

57 Rojter S, Santarelli MT, Albornoz L, Mastai R. Somatostatin in acute variceal bleeding: a meta-analysis study. *J Hepatol* 1993; **19**: 189–190.

58 Bernard B, Lebrec D, Mathurin P, Opolon P, Poynard T. Meta-analysis of beta-

blockers in the prevention of recurrent variceal bleeding in patients with cirrhosis. *Hepatology* 1994; **20**: 106A.

59 Fardy JM, Laupacis A. A meta-analysis of prophylactic endoscopic sclerotherapy for esophageal varices. *Am J Gastroenterol* 1994; **89**: 1938–1948.

60 Merkel, C, Morabito A. Adding beta-blockers to sclerotherapy in the prevention of variceal rebleeding: a meta-analysis assessment. *J Hepatol* 1994; **21**: 918–919.

61 Gøtzsche PC, Gjørup I, Bonnén H, Brahe NEB, Becker U, Burcharth F. Somatostatin vs. placebo in bleeding oesophageal varices. A randomized trial and a meta-analysis. *Br Med J* 1995; **310**: 1495–1498.

62 Heresbach D, Jacquelinet C, Jouel O, Chaperon J, Bretagne JF, Gosselin M. Secondary prophylaxis by sclerotherapy versus banding ligation for bleeding esopageal varices: meta-analysis of randomized clinical trials. *Gastroenterol Clin Biol* (in press).

63 Møller S, Sørensen TIA, Tygstrup N and the Copenhagen Esophageal Varices Sclerotherapy Project. Who benefits from endoscopic sclerotherapy of bleeding oesophageal varices? Proposal for differential indications. *J Hepatol* 1992; **15**: 184–191.

64 Calès P, Lacaine F, Bleichner G, Valla D, Lamouliatte H, Belghiti J, Bernades P. The emergency treatment of upper gastrointestinal bleeding due to portal hypertension in cirrhotic patients. Report on a French consensus meeting. *Eur J Gastroenterol Hepatol* 1991; **3**: 413–418.

65 Calès P, Oberti F. Stratégie du traitement hémostatique des hémorragies par rupture de varices oesophagiennes et gastriques. *Gastroenterol Clin Biol* (in press).

66 Paquet K-J, Kalk J-F, Klein C-P, Giad HA. Prophylactic sclerotherapy for esophageal varices in high risk cirrhotic patients selected by endoscopic and hemodynamic criteria: a randomized, single-center controlled trial. *Endoscopy* 1994; **26**: 734–740.

67 Bosch J, Garcia-Pagan JC, Feu F *et al.* New approaches in the pharmacologic treatment of portal hypertension. *J Hepatol* 1993; **17** (Suppl. 2): S41–S45.

68 The Standards of Reporting Trials Group. A proposal for structured reporting of randomized controlled trials. *JAMA* 1994; **272**: 1926–1931.

69 Gluud C, Sørensen TIA. New developments in the conduct and management of multicenter trials: an international review of clinical trial units. *Fundamental and Clinical Pharmacology* (in press).

Baveno II Consensus Statements: Trials in Portal Hypertension

Christian Gluud (Chairman), Ulrik Becker, Andrew K. Burroughs, Paul Calés, Alessandro Liberati, Alberto Morabito and Fabio Tiné

Strategy regarding randomized clinical trials

1 RCTs should meet Good Clinical Practice requirements.

2 RCTs should, if possible, register centrally. The Cochrane Collaboration could form the basis for such a register.

3 More powerful predictive factors associated with first variceal bleeding, continued bleeding and recurrent bleeding must be defined.

4 RCTs should have sufficient power, i.e. larger RCTs should be performed.

5 More powerful predictive variables of therapeutic response in relation to first variceal bleeding, continued bleeding and recurrent variceal bleeding must be defined.

6 RCTs should, if possible, include quality-of-life and health-economic assessments using appropriate methodology.

7 RCTs should include data on end-points on which there exist consensus.

8 RCTs should use structured reporting.

Strategy regarding meta-analyses

1 The Cochrane Collaboration offers an interesting opportunity in the field of portal hypertension as in other fields of medicine. An international Cochrane Collaborative Review Group dealing with treatment of bleeding varices and primary and secondary prophylaxis of bleeding varices should be formed.

2 All therapies should be monitored by cumulative meta-analyses in order to avoid unnecessary duplication.

3 Meta-analysis based on individual patient data could be performed in order to identify prognostic and therapeutic variables.

4 Complications, quality-of-life, and health-economic analysis should, if possible, be incorporated into the analyses of RCTs.

Index